INTERMITTENT FASTING FOR WOMEN

The complete guide to lose weight, reset metabolism, increase your energy and living healthy. Includes quick and easy recipes.

Nadia Wilmots

Copyright © 2021 by Nadia Wilmots. All rights reserved.

No part of this book may be reproduced or transmitted in any form or by any means, electronic or mechanical, including photocopying, recording or by information storage and retrieval system, without the written permission of the author.

Editing by Nadia Wilmots

Table of Contents

CHAPTER 1: INTRODUCTION 1
   INTERMITTENT FASTING IS BASED ON YEARS OF RESEARCH 3
   SOME FACTS ABOUT FASTING 3
   3. MEDICAL DISCOVERY OFTEN BEGINS WITH SELF-EXPERIMENT 4
   4. INTERMITTENT FASTING HELPS REDUCE FAT, NOT MUSCLE
   WHAT IS INTERMITTENT FASTING? 5
   HOW SHOULD IT BE? 6
CHAPTER 2: 8
ADVANTAGES OF FASTING 8
   ADVANTAGES 9
   PHYSIOLOGICAL BENEFITS 10
   LIFESTYLE BENEFITS 10
   PHYSICAL BENEFITS 15
   1. THE DECREASE IN BODY FAT 16
   2. CHOLESTEROL DEPOSITS ARE DECOMPOSED 16
   3. FIBRINOLYSIS 16
   4. ACCELERATION OF SELF-DECOMPOSITION 16
   5. INCREASED DIURESIS 16
   6. ACCELERATE PHAGOCYTOSIS 16
   FASTING GUIDELINES 17
   2. LEAN GAINS 17
   3. NATIONAL ASSEMBLY OF WARRIORS 17
   4. FAST EVERY OTHER DAY 18
   FACTS ABOUT INTERMITTENT FASTING 18
   FASTING AND BRAIN 18
   CAN FASTING MAKE YOU SMARTER? 20

CHAPTER 3: PURPOSE FOR STARTING 23
    ANTHROPOMETRY 28
    TAKE THE FOLLOWING MEASUREMENTS: 28
    BAND HISTORY 29
    INTERMITTENT FASTING AND DIET 30
    FAST IS YOUR FRIEND 30
CHAPTER 4: 32
KINDS OF FASTING 32
    MAHA-SHIVARATRI 32
    MEDICAL FASTING 32
    FASTING SCIENCE 33
    LENT 34
    SPIRITUAL FASTING 34
    RAMADAN 34
    FIVE INTERMITTENT FASTING VARIANTS 35
    FAST FOR 36 HOURS EVERY OTHER DAY / 12 HOURS 35
    EAT STOP EAT 24 HOURS QUICKLY, 1-2 TIMES AWEEK 36
    SKIPPING MEAL 36
    LEAN GAINS 16H FAST / 8H FEED - THIS IS THE FASTWE RECOMMEND IN OUR WORKSHOPS 36
    SO, WHAT ARE THE STEPS? 42
    2.   SELECT THE DISTRIBUTION OF FAST / MEALDETERMINE WHEN TO EAT AND FAST 42
    3.   SPEND A FLIRT DAY 43
    4.   TEACH PEOPLE 43
    5.   BUY BRANCHED-CHAIN AMINO ACIDS (OPTIONAL) 43
    6.   TRAINING AND INTERMITTENT FASTING 44
CHAPTER 5: 46
THE PROVOCATION OF INTERMITTENTFASTING 46
    BE CAREFUL AND EAT 46
    MENTAL FRAMEWORK 47

- LEVEL 1 BREATHE NATURALLY 48
- HAVE FUN 49
- JUNK FOOD 49
- LEVEL 2 CONTROLLED BREATHING 50
- LEVEL 3 VISUALIZE DISTRACTIONS 50
- LEVEL 4 INSTANT FOCUSES 51

CHAPTER 6: 53
WHEN WILL YOU START? 53
- LONG TERM EXPERIENCE 59
- FLEXIBILITY: THE KEY TO SUCCESS 59
- MAINTENANCE MODEL 59
- HOW YOUR ANATOMY CHANGES? 60
- FEMALE SPEED: MIMI'S EXPERIENCE 62
- 6 WAYS TO MAKE A FAST DIET EFFECTIVE 64
  - 2. FIND A QUICK FRIEND 65
  - 3. QUICK MEAL PREPARATION 66
  - 4. CHECK THE PARTIAL SIZE OF THE CALORIE LABEL ... 66
  - 5. STAY BUSY 67
  - 6. TRY 2 TO 2 67
- A TERRIBLE FAST FOR WOMEN? 67
- FASTING AND FUSSING 70
- CHOOSE THE RIGHT MEAL 70
- INGREDIENTS FOR HEALTHY FASTING-FOOD 71
- FASTING FUTURE: WHERE TO GO FROM HERE? 72
- STARTING INTERMITTENT FASTING YOUR FIRST 30 DAYS 74

CHAPTER 7: 78
SHOULD YOU FAST? 78
- LISTEN TO YOUR BODY 78
- FASTING AND DIABETES 79
- GET DOCTOR APPROVAL 79
- MANAGE CHRONIC ILLNESSES 79

- PREPARE FOR FASTING 80
- STARTING YOGA 81
- MAKE FASTING EASY 81

CHAPTER 8: 84
FAST DAY COOKING TIPS 84

- TIPS FOR A FAST DAY COOKING 84
- IMPROVED APPETITE 86
- TASTE AND INTERMITTENT FASTING 87
- FOOD TO RETHINK 89
- HOW TO CHOOSE ZERO-DAY? 91
- DAILY SWITCHING 94
- DAILY STRATEGY 94
- WHAT TO EAT? 95
  2. ADD WATER 96
  3. DO NOT EXPECT WEIGHT LOSS ON ANYPARTICULAR DAY 96
  4. BE WISE, BE CAREFUL, AND STOP IF YOU FEELWRONG..... 96
  5. CONGRATULATIONS 97
- HOW ABOUT ALCOHOL? 98
- AND CAFFEINE? 98
- SHAKE/JUICE? 99
- WHO ELSE SHOULD NOT FAST? 100
- DO YOU HAVE A HEADACHE? 101
- DO YOU HAVE TO WORRY ABOUT HYPOGLYCEMIA? 101
- I'M TIRED !!! 101
- HOWEVER, DO I SLEEP HUNGRY? 102
- WILL, MY BODY GO INTO HUNGER MODE ANDCONTINUES TO GET FAT? 102
- WHAT IF EVERYONE AROUND ME EATS ONE OF MYFASTING DAYS? 102
- WHAT IF I AM CURRENTLY OBESE? 103

CONCLUSION 105

DELICIOUS RECIPES 107
   SPICY CHOCOLATE FAT BOMBS 107
   AVOCADO QUESADILLAS 109
   COBB SALAD WITH BROWN DERBY DRESSING 111
   LEMON SALMON 113
   VEGGIE CHEESY CHICKEN SALAD 115
   FRIED 'FISH' TACOS 117
   TILAPIA PARMESAN 120
   CHICKEN BREASTS WITH AVOCADO TAPENADE 122
   ROASTED BROCCOLI W LEMON GARLIC & PINE NUTS 124
   BRUSSELS SPROUTS WITH BACON AND ONIONS 126
   BAKED POTATO 128
   CAULIFLOWER POPCORN 130
   LENTIL BURGERS 132
   BLACK BEAN SOUP 134
   SAUERKRAUT SALAD 136
   COCONUT KEFIR BANANA MUFFINS 138

CHAPTER 1:

INTRODUCTION

Eating habits have disappeared in recent decades, but the usual medical advice for a healthy lifestyle remains the same: eat low-fat foods, get more exercise than skipping meals. Over the same period, obesity skyrocketed worldwide. So, is there another evidence-based approach that depends on science, not opinion? When we first read the supposed benefits of intermittent fasting, we were as skeptical as others. Fasting appeared intense and challenging. We knew that diets were usually doomed to failure, although both were described. But we did thorough research and tested it ourselves, so we are convinced of its tremendous potential. One of the doctors interviewed for this book said, "Do nothing to your body that is as strong as fasting."

It was developed at a time when there was a shortage of food. We have been the product of festivals and famines for thousands of years. The reason we respond so well to intermittent fasting is that it mimics the environment in which modern humans train much more closely than three meals a day. Of course, fasting is a product of faith for many. Lent, Yom Kippur, and Ramadan are just a few of the most common examples. Greek Orthodox Christians are advised to fast 180 days a year (according to Saint Nicholas of Zicha, an overabundance makes a dark and anxious man, but a fast makes him happy and brave), Buddhist monks fast every month on the moon. But many of us seem to be eating most of the time. We are rarely hungry. But we are not satisfied with our weight, our body, and our health. Intermittent fasting can bring us back into contact with humans. It is not only for weight loss but also for long-term health and well-being. Scientists are just beginning to discover and demonstrate the power of a tool. This book is the result of his cutting-edge research and his impact on current thinking on weight loss, disease resistance, and longevity.

But it is also the result of our personal experience. Here, we study intermittent fasting from two complementary angles, because the laboratory and the lifestyle are relevant. First, using physical and medical training to test his potential, Michael explained the science behind intermittent fasting and the 5: 2 diets, and caught the world's eye last summer. The context and history of the fast made it possible to understand the process.

Fasting: old ideas, modern methods. Fasting is not new. Your body is designed to fast, as you will learn in the next chapter.

INTERMITTENT FASTING IS BASED ON YEARS OF RESEARCH

Animal fasting research dates back 80 years. Research on human fasting goes back at least six years. More and more clinical studies are underway for research.

In an early 1945 study, mice were fasted for four days, one day, three days, or two days. Researchers have found that fasted mice live longer. They also found that fasted mice were not physically stunted, unlike calorie-depleted mice. Since then, at least in rodents, the value of fasting has been confirmed in numerous studies. But why is fasting useful? What is the mechanism?

Valter has access to his supply of transgenic mice called dwarf or Laron mice. These mice, although small, hold records of the extended lifespan of mammals. In other words, they have lived surprisingly long. The average mouse has a modest lifespan, probably two years. Laron mice last twice as long, and many have a calorie restriction for more than four years. In humans, this equates to almost 170 years. What makes the Laron mouse attractive is the fact that it not only has a long lifespan, but it also keeps most of its life very long through opting the intermittent fastings. They just seem less prone to diabetes and cancer, which is a natural cause when they die. Valter told me that autopsy often fails to find the cause of death. They just seem dead.

SOME FACTS ABOUT FASTING

2. HUNGER MODE

Studies that demonstrated the adverse effects of fasting

were done in the 1950s. In this study, they took several young men and asked them to live on about half their regular calories. They tracked for six months, apparently losing weight dramatically. There was a severe problem when her body fat dropped to 5%. Well, it is radically fast for a long time. There was no excellent structure in this attempt, and weight loss was completed too early. It has led to adverse health problems. Intermittent fasting is not like that.

3. MEDICAL DISCOVERY OFTEN BEGINS WITH SELF-EXPERIMENT

Until you try it, you are not sure how fasting can help. Everyone is different, everyone is unique, and it is essential to monitor it. What works for others cannot work for you. If your fasts do not work, try another one.

4. INTERMITTENT FASTING HELPS REDUCE FAT, NOTMUSCLE

Fasting speeds up your metabolism, resets your digestive system, and activates your metabolism.

Fasting promotes longevity - studies have shown how the lives of people in certain cultures have improved as a result of their diet.

Fasting improves hunger - it takes 12 to 24 hours to feel the real need. You will notice this when you are fasting.

Fasting improves your brain function - because it increases the production of a protein called the Brain-Derived Neurotrophic Factor (BDNF).

Fasting improves your immune system - because it reduces free radical damage, regulates inflammation in the body, and stops cancer cells from forming. When you are sick, your instinct is to focus on resting rather than eating.

Fasting helps to clean the skin and prevent acne. It is because the temporarily undigested body can concentrate its regenerative energy on other systems.

WHAT IS INTERMITTENT FASTING?

What exactly does intermittent fasting refer to? Almost all of usare familiar with the word fasting. The reasons people fast vary from one group to another.
For some, it is a religious practice; they sacrifice food to commit to prayer. Others have no reason; they just lack food. In past societies, people would go out to the fields to work, and eat only when they rested.
Intermittent fasting is not among the fasting practices described above. It is neither a religious practice, nor is it driven by the lack of time or food - it is a choice. It is best described as an eating pattern that alternates between eating periods and fasting periods, with each period lasting a predetermined amount of time. For example, the 16:8 method has a fasting period of 16 hours and an eating period of 8 hours.
Note that it is not a diet but an eating pattern. Less is said about the foods you should eat, but more emphasis is put on when you eat them.
Does this mean you can eat whatever you want? Unfortunately not. Just like anything else in life, you're going to get out what you put in.
Clean eating is one of the three factors in the tripod to fat burning success. Does this mean you must live on chicken

and broccoli? No of course not. We are humans and I believe in

enjoying life, but as you already know moderation is the key here.

It is important to know that IF isn't some program that popped up from somewhere, will trend for a while, and disappear like most weight loss programs do. It has been around for a long time and has been popular for many years (even if you are learning about it just now). It is one of the leading health and fitness trends in the world today.

It is recommended by a range of health and fitness experts, let us learn more about how intermittent fasting works in the following chapter.

HOW SHOULD IT BE?

Let us dive into the "heart of the problem" by providing you with some idea of why and how intermittent fasting should be considered. Intermittent fasting allows you to structure and work towards your aspirations; for example, weight loss, we find that fewer calories consumed are correlated with weight loss. During your fasting period, the calorie intake is significantly reduced because the time window for eating has also decreased. The phenomenon encourages better adaptability to insulin secretion of the growth hormone, two essential components for losing weight and muscle profit. This practice will not only help you lose weight but also maintain your weight, which is the path to your goal. During the process, you will notice how everything comes into perspective. You will realize that not only your weight loss goal is achieved, but your other goals as well by seeing how your daily tasks and behaviors become simpler. The process eliminates the need for food preparations (what, when, and where to eat). Which could inevitably save you more of your reduced diet?! Now you have time to focus on other activities instead of contemplating at three or more meals a day; the 16/8 method only requires preparing two meals. This method now allows you to enjoy more substantial portions of your time. You are causing the stomach and taste buds to fill up while consuming simultaneously fewer calories.

CHAPTER 2:

ADVANTAGES OF FASTING

Do you want to lose fat, build muscle, gain energy, and feel like a new person simply and sustainably? And do you need a diet-free approach that delivers results at significantly accelerated rates? Now let me introduce you to intermittent fasting - the most sustainable and most comfortable fitness trick to get you into the best shape of your life. Intermittent fasting has grown in popularity over the past year, as its benefits and consequences have become apparent. You were used by celebrities like Hugh Jackman, Beyonce, Benedict Cumber batch, and Ben Affleck. This book is short and deliberate. I want you to act, and you haven't sat and read books for hours. Knowledge is not power but potential power. Power comes from the implementation of experience. And that is what intermittent fasting is. To precisely convey the knowledge, you need to perform actions and display results and to achieve excellent results. Now let us practice the simple habit of intermittent fasting to get the best shape of your life. Well, it is not a diet; it is a new approach to eating. Intermittent fasting is a cyclical process of eating along with the periods you are not eating. These short fasting periods cause various hormonal reactions in your body. These answers lead to incredible benefits and results.

ADVANTAGES

Here are some examples (do not diet or restrict foods that you can eat)

- Increase muscle mass quickly
- Increase in energy level
- Increased production of testosterone and growth hormone
- Improve cognitive function

Fasting is the most effective way to stay fit and well, as fasting is based on scientific knowledge, not "bro-science."

If you are in good shape and have failed, do not despair. The problem with most diets is that you place too many restrictions on what you can eat. Intermittent fasting is the opposite-you do not have to make any changes to your diet to earn rewards.

So, what are you waiting for? Immerse yourself in the book now and learn everything you need to know about intermittent fasting. We will walk you through each step and provide a simple, easy-to-follow guide to get the results you have always wanted.

I think that the popularity of IF is increasing mainly due to the following two factors.

- An extensive list of significant benefits.
- Easy acceptance and maintenance.

It is essential because it has been shown that most diets and diet plans fail due to the two main obstacles. These obstacles are the complexity of managing nutrition and the time it takes to demonstrate results. How many times do you think "eating this food negatively affects my diet"? or "I eat XYZ in 2 weeks, but I cannot get the results I expected". Have you heard Intermittent fasting cleanly breaks through these barriers due to their simple and straightforward procedure and the speed with which they arise? The IF concept contradicts many of the longstanding beliefs of the fitness and health industries, but as this book describes in detail, something is popularized by everyone and their grandmother, and this does not mean it is true. Prevailing myths of fitness and nutrition Intermittent fasts underwent extensive tests at the start of their emergence, as they violate everything that has been taught in the fitness industry for the past 50 years. At first glance, the concept of deliberately not eating is a fitness error. However, by exploring your ideas and using scientific data to challenge past assumptions, you will find shocking things.

PHYSIOLOGICAL BENEFITS

- Rapid Fat Loss
- Increase in Testosterone and HGH Production
- Lean Muscle Gain
- Increased Energy Levels
- Ability to Easily Control Hunger
- Higher Sex Drive
- Improvement to Hair and Skin
- Longevity of Life

LIFESTYLE BENEFITS

- Improvement of cognitive capacity
- Better sleep
- Win time and money
- Easy to follow

- Reduction of stress

Therefore, intermittent fasting has many benefits that make it the perfect way to lose fat, build muscle and feel good. One of the main factors behind the ability of FI to burn fat quickly is that when the body is starved, the body attacks the fat to start providing energy. Another way for IFs to lose weight fast is to cut calories in the diet simply. By changing the time to eat and reducing the amount of time you can eat naturally, you will reduce the number of calories you eat, and this will start to shed unnecessary body fat. Fasting also increases the oxidation of fatty acids, which in turn speeds up the fat-burning process. It allows your body to burn fat at high levels during and after the fast. Many hormonal reactions also occur when the body is fasting. One of the primary responses is that growth hormone and testosterone begin to be secreted by the body is considerably increased amounts. How significant is the increase? In one study, another point that I want to explain is that fasting also reduces the production of the hormone ghrelin. It is a hormone that affects hunger and satiety. If you've ever suffered from hunger, ghrelin has been produced more. When it is sober, it becomes dull and effectively prevents the feeling of hunger when fasting. As I mentioned at the beginning of the book, fasting is not a diet but a diet. For me, this is one of the most important advantages. It is easy to follow, suitable for all lifestyles, and you can enjoy all of its significant benefits without disturbing your social life. Eating is beneficial and religiously very practical, but this is often difficult because many foods are prohibited. Have you ever been on a diet with your friends? It is stupid to find something on the menu. Remove intermittent fasting as it does not benefit from the food you eat, but from the physiological reactions that cause it. Following specific nutritional guidelines (discussed later) will, of course, speed up your results, but the critical point is that you do not have to eat the same meal more than once. Intermittent fasting style In the IF world, you can use different methods.

Thirty-six hours quickly once every 8-10 days. Only well-trained intermittent accelerations. The 36-hour speed is a mental struggle to be overcome. The benefits are enormous but challenging to complete and to challenge to integrate into your lifestyle. Do not exceed 36 hours as your body burns all your fat reserves and starts attacking your muscles for energy. The final meal / fast time you choose does not significantly affect your goals, as each option offers the desired benefits. However, what matters is consistency in respecting the options you want. If you like it, do not do it by accident. To get results and benefits, you must continuously adhere to fasting times. You do not have to stick to the same meals and fasts every day, but sticking to them is much more comfortable. It is a lifestyle, not a diet.

Each class has advantages and disadvantages, but both have the miracles described in the previous chapter. The effect of benefits will vary slightly between individual options. Therefore, choosing the style that best suits your lifestyle is paramount. All IF techniques revolve around the same basic concept. In other words, a large fasting window and a small dining room window. The most common fasting meals/hours are 16 divisions. Each day consists of 16 hours of fasting, followed by 8 hours of meals. It is the simplest to adopt, and it is recommended for beginners. If you sleep about half the time, hiring is very easy.

Division 18/6. Each day consists of an 18 hour fast followed by a 6-hour meal window. After 6 p.m., the fasting effect increased significantly, speeding up the results of the 4 p.m. window. It is recommended to do this after experiencing the 16/8 division. In division 20/4, each day consists of 20 hours of fasting, followed by 4 hours of meals. I think it is a convenient window, but it is as fast as 20 hours a day, so it is tough to avoid this effect-24 hour quickly. It takes place twice a week. Once you have that, it is not for beginners to have experience with various fasting windows, so you can jump to it, but do not try it as a beginner. Beginners who try to fast for 24 hours often fail because they are not yet used to fasting.

In this chapter, I would like to deepen this concept. First, let's see what defines a meal in the dictionary. "A selection of certain foods that have been developed or prescribed to improve a person's physical condition, such preference or limitation of the amount a person eats to lose weight that of a specific person or group food is consumed. "When I read these sentences, I only see the limit - it is about eating in my head. You set too many restrictions on what you can eat and how much you can eat, and everything is more confusing than it should be. Now I would like to point out that a diet can be beneficial, but I find it very specific for a purpose (such as achieving single-digit body fat percentage) or for medical reasons. For most people, the diet is not sufficient, but it does not give the desired results and has a massive failure rate. The plans are limited. Intermittent fasting is not limiting; it frees you from all the technical details of the project. When you start exercising when you do not have to stick to incredibly strict dietary rules, instead, you can eat what you want (with reason) and more (with reason again). Eating fast food every day makes sense as if you are eating ridiculous, and drugs, fitness routines, and supplements will not help you lose weight and lose weight. Fast food is harmful to health, harms hormones, the brain, and internal organs.

Intermittent fasting is different from the diet because the food rules do not bound it. Do you want to eat white carbohydrates? You are welcome! Do you want a pizza for tonight? You are welcome! Do you not wish to change your current dining style? Well, it is the answer. If you are going to go one step further and see significantly accelerated results and more significant benefits, you can make specific nutritional choices. Accelerate results with food As I mentioned earlier, the primary use of IF is the hormonal response that occurs when your body is fasting. However, you can speed up your results by changing your current eating style and following certain principles. Following these guidelines and regulations will speed up your results when you eat foods such as:

- Increases the production of testosterone and growth hormone
- Helps burn fat
- Reduces insulin spikes
- Helps in muscle growth
- Improves cognitive function
- So, if you are looking for accelerated results, here are the guidelines that I follow.
- Avoid processed and manufactured foods
- Avoid white carbohydrates
- Increase the amount of protein in your diet

- Increase the number of healthy fats in your diet (olive oil, avocado, etc.)
- Make sure 80% of the carbohydrates come from legumes and beans
- Make sure the remaining 20% of carbohydrates come from whole grains and whole wheat
- Eat green vegetables with each meal
- Use the following seasoning: garlic, pepper, cayenne pepper, chili flakes, black pepper, sea salt.
- Reduce fruit consumption and limit yourself to 1 fruit per day
- Drink only black coffee, herbal tea, and water

Again, you do not have to follow these guidelines, but if you follow them, your results and benefits will be accelerated. Now you've read all about IF and understand how powerful it is. We recommend that you read this chapter rather than fasting. Before you start practicing FI, I suggest some steps. The information here will help your neurotrophic factor (BDNF).

PHYSICAL BENEFITS

Fasting improves your immune system - because it reduces free radical damage, regulates inflammation in the body, and stops cancer cells from forming. When you are sick, your instinct is to focus on resting rather than eating. Fasting helps to clean the skin and prevent acne. This is because the temporarily undigested body can concentrate its regenerative energy on other systems.

Body reaction when stopping

The following happens to your body during a fast:

1. THE DECREASE IN BODY FAT

It leads to weight loss and helps reduce the risk of heart disease, stroke, cancer, diabetes, etc.

2. CHOLESTEROL DEPOSITS ARE DECOMPOSED

When you are hungry, remove waste quickly. Cholesterol usually includes cholesterol stored in the inner lining of blood vessels. Cholesterol levels may increase in the first week after fasting when the body detoxifies, but they decrease.

3. FIBRINOLYSIS

Dangerous blood clots that accumulate in the body are easily broken down on an empty stomach. This process is called fibrinolysis.

4. ACCELERATION OF SELF-DECOMPOSITION

Every cell in the body contains its seed of destruction. When it needs itself, the section releases its self-destructing enzymes and self

Destruction. That is self-decomposition. During fasting, this type of tissue is destroyed during the process of autolysis, affecting normal function.

5. INCREASED DIURESIS

Diuresis is the excretion from the kidney. During the fast, the body voluntarily and automatically eliminates salt and water without damaging the tissues of the body. This diuresis has enormous health benefits.

6. ACCELERATE PHAGOCYTOSIS

During the rapid defense of white blood cells, they

destroy toxic bacteria and accelerate their ability to digest waste products. White blood cells of fasted people were very effective in killing toxic bacteria. Below are the four most popular fasting style guides. This list is not exhaustive and covers only the most popular, but it will undoubtedly give you an idea of your goals. Below you will find the four most popular fasting style guides. This list is not extensive and only covers the most popular, but it will certainly give you some thoughts about your goals.

FASTING GUIDELINES

1. REGULARLY FAST (EAT STOP EAT)

This is usually a 24-hour speed that you will pace periodically. You can start this at any time of the day and do it once or twice a week. This type of fasting is sifted through by Brad Pyron, and it is recommended to fast for 24 hours every 3-5 days to lose weight.

2. LEAN GAINS

Use this method to fast for 16 hours at a time, for example, from 10 p.m. to 2 p.m. After that, three meals are taken in the remaining 8 hours. Martin Berkhan wrote lean gains, and the plan also includes details about the movement. So, if you want to fast and continue exercising, this could be your plan.

3. NATIONAL ASSEMBLY OF WARRIORS

This is just a step away from lean gains. This method only promotes one healthy meal a day (usually dinner). Research by State et al. Let's take a closer look at that. In this study, familiar weight participants used enough energy to maintain the weight of one meal or three meals a day for eight weeks. Despite the same calorie consumption, participants lost weight between one meal a day and three meals a day. Fat mass was significantly reduced, and muscle mass tended to increase after eating one meal a day for eight weeks. However, during the 8-week study period, hunger increased steadily with just one meal a day, suggesting that appetite hormones were not adjusting.

4. FAST EVERY OTHER DAY

This is an intermittent fasting style. Food is consumed for 24 hours and is restricted the next day—Heilbronn etc. We conducted a detailed survey on this. The study was conducted on eight healthy-weight men and eight women who fasted every 21 days. Participants lost approximately $2.5 \pm 0.5\%$ of body weight, including $4 \pm 1\%$ of fat, over 21 days. The fasting blood sugar and ghrelin (appetite hormone) levels did not change before and after the procedure. Still, the fasting insulin level was low, indicating a high level of insulin sensitivity. Studies also showed that the metabolic machinery needed to generate energy from fat was sufficient at the start of the course.

FACTS ABOUT INTERMITTENT FASTING

Here are some facts about intermittent fasting you may not know, but you should know before you start. Most of the initial long-term studies on the benefits of fasting are done in rodents. They also gave us valuable insights into the molecular mechanisms underlying fasting.

FASTING AND BRAIN

As Woody Allen once said, the brain is my second favorite organ. Nothing else would work without them so that

I could put it first. The human brain, about three pounds of a pinkish-grey exaggeration, is Tapioca's constant object, which is described as the most complex object in the known universe. It enables us to build, write poems, rule the planet, and understand ourselves. It is also a very efficient energy-saving machine that does all this intricate work and makes sure your body is working correctly while using the same amount of energy as a 25-watt bulb. The fact that our brains are usually very flexible and adaptable makes it even more tragic when they go wrong. I know that as I grow older, my memory becomes more error-prone. I've supplemented it with various memory tips I've learned over the years, but I'm still having trouble remembering names and dates. But much worse than that, is the fear that one day I may completely lose my head and probably develop some form of dementia. I want to keep my brain in the best possible condition and keep it as long as possible. Fortunately, fasting seems to provide the necessary protection.

It was Professor Mark Mattson who talked about the brain. Mark Mattson, a professor of neuroscience at the National Institute for Aging, is one of the most respected scientists in his field, researching the aged brain. I find his work exciting - which suggests that fasting can help fight diseases like Alzheimer's, dementia, and memory loss. I could have taken a taxi to his office, but I wanted to go. I like to go for a walk. Not only does it burn calories, but it also improves one's mood and helps to keep your memory. Although the brain shrinks typically with age, a study found that in everyday pedestrians, the hippocampus, an area of the brain essential for memory, is enlarged compared to that of the mind of a seated person. Mark, who studies

Alzheimer's disease, lost his father to dementia. He was not willing to work directly on this area of research, but when he started working on Alzheimer's disease, he told me that his father had not been diagnosed, so he provided insight.

Alzheimer's disease affects approximately 26 million people worldwide, and the problems increase with the aging of the population. The tragedy of Alzheimer's disease and other forms of dementia can delay, but cannot prevent, unavoidable deterioration after diagnosis, so a new approach is urgently needed. You can get worse and worse until you need years of ongoing care. After all, you may not even notice the faces of those you once loved.

CAN FASTING MAKE YOU SMARTER?

Marc took me to see mice, as Valter Longo did. Like Valter's mouse, Mark's mouse is genetically modified but modified to be more vulnerable to Alzheimer's disease. The rat I saw was in a maze and had to navigate to find food. Some mice do this relatively quickly. Others are confused and confused. This task and others are designed to reveal signs of memory impairment in mice. A struggling mouse quickly forgets which arm of the maze has already gone down.

Genetically modified mice with Alzheimer's disease develop dementia as soon as they take a regular diet. By the time they are one year old, they represent the average human age, and they usually have evident learning and memory problems. Animals continue to fast intermittently. Mark calls this "intermittent energy limitation" and is often up to 20 months without any signs of dementia 9. They do not start to get worse until the end of their lives. In humans, it is the same as the signs of Alzheimer's disease appearing at age 80 rather than age 50. I know which one I prefer. Worryingly, these mice descend much faster than a normal-fed mouse on a regular junk food diet. "We fed mice a diet high in fat and fructose," Mark said, and "this has a dramatic effect. We have a lot of problems accumulating a lot of amyloids and finding ways in the maze test." In other words, junk food makes these mice fat and stupid.

One of the most significant changes that occur in Mark's hungry mouse brain is the increased production of a protein called the neurotrophic factor from the brain. BDNF has been shown to stimulate stem cells into new neurons in the hippocampus. As mentioned earlier, this is a part of the brain that is essential for everyday learning and memory. But why does the hippocampus grow in response to hunger? Mark points out that it makes sense from an evolutionary perspective. After all, you have to be smarter and, on the ball, if you do not have a lot to eat. "When animals are in areas with limited food resources, it is essential to remember where the feed is, where it is at risk, predators, etc. I think people in the past have had a survival advantage."

It is not known precisely whether new brain cells will develop in response to a fast. To be sure, researchers need to intermittently fast and kill volunteers, remove the brain, and look for new signs of nerve growth. Many people rarely volunteer for such projects. But what they are doing is a study that uses volunteers immediately and then MRI to see if their hippocampal size changes over time. As mentioned earlier, these techniques are used in humans to show that regular exercise, such as walking increases the size of the hippocampus. Hopefully, similar studies show that intermittent fasting two days a week is good for learning and memory. On a purely anecdotal level, using a sample size of 1 seems to work. Before I started the fast diet, I did an ingenious memory test online. After two months of testing, performance improved.

CHAPTER 3:

PURPOSE FOR STARTING

What does not kill us makes us stronger!? Several researchers influenced me in various ways, but the one who stands out is Professor Mark Mattson of the National Institute for Aging in Baltimore. A few years ago, she wrote an article with Edward Scalabrese in New Scientist magazine, "When a little poison is good for you."

"Small poison is good for you" is a colorful way of explaining the theory of Hermes's: the idea that humans and other creatures can be enhanced when they are exposed to stress and toxins. Hermes is not just a variant that "if you join the army, you become a man." It is now the accepted biology explanation of how things work at the cellular level. For example, consider something as simple as exercising. When you run or pump iron, it damages your muscles and causes minor wear & tears. If it is not thoroughly exceeded, your body will respond with repairs, strengthening your muscles.

Vegetables are another example. We all know that fruits and vegetables are full of antioxidants, so you should eat a lot.

The problem with this generally accepted explanation of how fruits and vegetables "work" is that they are probably wrong or at least incomplete. The level of antioxidants in fruits and vegetables is shallow and obviously cannot have the profound effects they have. Furthermore, attempts to extract antioxidants from plants and provide us in concentrated form as a health-promoting supplement were not convincing in long-term trials. Beta-carotene is suitable for you if taken in the way of carrots. When they took beta carotene from carrots and administered it as a supplement for cancer patients, it seemed to make them worse. By looking at how vegetables work in our bodies through the lens of Hermes's, we see that the reasons for their benefits can be very different.

Consider this apparent paradox. Bitterness is often associated with poison in nature and should be avoided. Plants produce a wide variety of so-called phytochemicals, some of which act as natural pesticides to keep mammals like us from eating them. The fact that they taste bitter is a clear warning sign: stay away. So, there is an evolutionary reason why we should not love ourselves and avoid bitter-tasting foods. However, even as adults, many of us find it hard to love them because some of the vegetables that are particularly good for us, such as cabbage, cauliflower, broccoli, and other members of the family of crucifers, are so bitter.

The solution to this paradox is that these vegetables are bitter because they contain chemicals that can be toxic. The reason they do not harm us is that these chemicals are contained in low, non-toxic doses. Instead, they activate the stress response and activate the genes that protect and repair.

Valter has been studying fasting for many years and is a determined believer. He is far from research, following a low-protein, vegetable-rich diet that his grandparents cherish in southern Italy. Perhaps not coincidentally, her grandparents live in parts of Italy where people are highly concentrated in the long run. In addition to a reasonably strict diet, Valter skips lunch and loses weight. Beyond that, once every six months, he has an extended fast that lasts for several days. Tall, slim, energetic, and Italian, he is an inspiring poster designer for future fasts. The main reason he is so interested in fasting is that his and other studies have shown an exceptional array of measurable health benefits that you get from it. As he explained, many "repair genes" can be activated and bring long-term benefits, even without a short-term diet, he explained. "There is a lot of early evidence that temporary fasting can lead to permanent changes that can have a positive effect on aging and illness," he told me. "You take people; you fast them. After 24 hours, everything is revolutionary. And even if you take a cocktail of drugs, a potent drug, you will never get closer. The nice thing about fasting is that everything is fine."

"To maintain a metabolic burn, you need to eat a small meal 5 to 6 times a day."

Unless you have lived under a rock in the past 20 years, I'm sure you've heard of it. It spreads like wildfire and is one of those few pieces of advice that everyone accepts. This advice is prevalent and is nearly taken for granted.

However, this is a lie without scientific evidence. Yes, one of the best fitness and health tips is wrong. The logic behind this theory is that a small meal during the day will burn more fat. This is based on the idea that if you eat frequently, your metabolism will increase as your metabolism increases. Unfortunately, this has not been proven, but many studies have tried and failed. As always, in scientific research, some groups try to prove the theory, and others try to deny it. The teams that refute it have won thanks to this prevalent theory of diet. Several articles have been published on the subject. The best known is the article entitled.

"We cannot lose weight by increasing the frequency of meals."

A team of Canadian researchers refuted the frequent eating pattern and said that the frequency, but the frequency, was not necessary.

I would point out here that you can lose weight with six small meals, but the reason for the weight loss is not the frequency or timing of the meals. Breakfast is the most important meal of the day. This sounds perfectly logical and has some inherent advantages, but not always, and there is plenty of evidence to deny this. I am not saying that breakfast is terrible or wrong or should be avoided. Just be aware that just being famous is not fair and that there are more effective strategies. The concept that breakfast is the most important meal of the day is that it helps you start the day, energizes you, and nourishes the day. You should keep in mind that most people make bad decisions at breakfast because these points are worth it for you. These decisions are the opposite of the expected benefits. In connection with this, the idea that eating food (especially carbohydrates) increases fat late in the evening - this is another common myth that science is debating. Subsequent feeding can lead to some of the following benefits: less fat, more testosterone, more sleep, and more muscles. There are advantages to not eating late at night, but there are indications that the benefits of eating later outweigh the benefits of eating early. If the practitioner recommends skipping breakfast, we will go into more detail then.

Another essential requirement for fitness and nutrition is that you need to eat certain foods and follow specific diets to achieve your goals. It does not matter if your goal is to lose weight, build muscle, or live longer and healthier lives, every guru, dietitian, and personal trainer uses their favorite diet as the only way to reach that goal.

Some of the everyday meals that you could follow are:

- Low in carbohydrates, high in protein, free of fat
- High fat and high protein content without carbohydrates
- Slow carbohydrate diet
- A DASH diet
- Paleolithic
- Bike cycling
- Atkins

There are hundreds of different diets that you can follow. Each has its strengths and weaknesses, but often all are lacking in one area. Of course, each of these diets can help you reach your goals, but no matter how effective your diet is, religious practice can hurt your progress. If you focus on a diet, limit your choices, and make it very difficult to follow. This leads to diet failure. Intermittent fasts avoid this because it does not promote a particular diet but suggest changes in the frequency and window of the diet. Yes, there are certain guidelines that you should follow, but they are very loose, and in most cases, you can eat whatever type of food you like. Before and after before after. Instead, take "before" and "after" (or "progress") photos. You can later compare them side by side to see how your body has changed over time. Photos can be a motivating tool because you may not notice the small changes that occur every day when you look at them. Make sure that your current dissatisfaction with your body does not prevent you from taking "front" pictures. They would be happy if they were on the go.

ANTHROPOMETRY

Anthropometry is helpful. You can start building muscle, especially if you exercise or do strength training regularly. When your body begins to change, you may not notice a significant change in scale, but your body composition can change dramatically. Measurements help you track your progress by monitoring the inches lost from different areas of your body.

TAKE THE FOLLOWING MEASUREMENTS:

•**Bust:** attach the measuring tape to the nipple and measure the entire breast.

•**Chest:** measurement: Measure directly under the chest or chest muscles and around the back.

•**Hips:** Find the widest part of your hips and measure your entire circumference.

•**Knee:** Measure up to just above the knee while standing upright.

- **Forearm:** Measures the entire forearm under the elbow.

- **Thigh:** Measure the whole thigh while standing upright.

- **Upper arm:** Measures the whole upper arm from the elbow.

- **Waist:** Find the narrowest part of your waist (usually just under your chest) and measure your entire circumference.

BAND HISTORY

For correct measurement, a measuring tape without elasticity is required. Hold the tape straight around your body and parallel to the floor. When making measurements, wrap the tape as close to the skin as possible, but do not squeeze the tape measure into the skin or squeeze it hard enough to create an indentation. It is helpful for someone else to take your measurements for you and allow you to stand straight. If no one is doing it, measure in front of the mirror and make sure the tape is held straight and in the right place.

Create a list of readings in your notebook or mobile phone notepad. Take measurements every few weeks and write down the numbers in the same place each time. You can use the measures to record your progress over time.

There are ups and downs. Like everything in life, you experience intermittent fasting, mostly ups and downs at the beginning. Do not expect everything to go smoothly from the front or be wholly absorbed in it. You glide as you will sometimes eat outside your feeding window, and it is okay. If you know you'll do your best, but you know that it can take some time to get used to the transition, you are less likely to be overwhelmed if your plan isn't on track.

INTERMITTENT FASTING AND DIET

Studies show that people who follow a nutritional plan tolerate variations in food choices such as intermittent fasting, eat more than the people on a strict calorie-controlled diet, more likely to stick, and maintain weight loss. A rigid diet is also associated with symptoms of eating disorders and a higher body mass index (a measure of body fat based on weight and height).

In the case of IF, even if you agree with the theory that the way to lose weight is to reduce calories and do more exercise, "you do not have to count calories, overeat, or avoid healthy fats," it is the good news.

FAST IS YOUR FRIEND

The benefits of fasting cover every aspect of your health, both physically and mentally. If you do it responsibly and carefully, it can help you control your body and well-being. There are many options for intermittent fasting. You need to choose a method that works best for you and helps you reach your health goals. We sometimes combine and experiment with techniques until we find one that we can commit to fasting and a healthy lifestyle.

One of the most common reasons people fast sometimes is weight loss, but it barely scratches the surface. Intermittent fasting does more to your body than helping you to lose weight. It also stabilizes blood sugar levels, relieves chronic or widespread inflammation, and improves heart health. Studies also show that intermittent fasting contributes to brain health and helps reduce the risk of developing severe brain disorders such as Alzheimer's disease. Finally, some researchers have proposed that it can help prevent cancer and improve the effectiveness of chemotherapy for people suffering from the disease.

CHAPTER 4:

KINDS OF FASTING

MAHA-SHIVARATRI

Hinduism is believed to deny the physical needs of the body through fasting to increase spirituality. Although fasting is an integral part of the Hindu religion and is practiced frequently, one of the most popular Fasting is during Maha-Shivaratri or the "Great Night of Shiva." During Maha-Shivaratri, the followers fast, participate in ritual baths, visit a temple where they pray, and practice the virtues of honesty, forgiveness, and self-discipline.

There are many reasons for fasting in Judaism, including asking for God's mercy, marking important life events, thanking God or praying to get out of grief; however, if you fast, it is common to keep the fasts private.

MEDICAL FASTING

Hippocrates, known as the "father of medicine," fasted during the 5th century BC as a medical therapy for some of his sick patients. One of the famous quotes from Hippocrates says, *"If you are sick, you eat your disease."* He believed that fasting allows the body to focus on healing and that forcing food into a sick state could harm your health because instead of giving energy for recovery, whatever was available energy, your body would consume indigestion. On the other hand, if sick patients abstain from eating, the digestive processes are interrupted, and the body would give priority to natural healing.

FASTING SCIENCE

Intermittent fasting has been accused of being a temporary epidemic, as have other nutritional concepts that take precedence over the health and diet communities. Still, the science behind the benefits of fasting is already growing. There are several theories as to why intermittent fasting works well, but the most frequently studied and most proven advantage is stress.

The word stress has different definitions, but to some emphasis, it is right for your health. For example, exercise is technically physical stress (mostly the muscle and cardiovascular system). Still, this stress ultimately strengthens your body as long as you have adequate recovery times in your daily life.

According to Dr. Mark Mattson, Principal Investigator and Director of the Institute for Neuroscience, National Institute for Aging, Professor of Neuroscience, Johns Hopkins University School of Medicine, intermittent fasting is a movement. Refusing food to the body for a defined period puts a small amount of stress on the cells. Over time, cells adapt to this stress by learning to manage it well. Your body's ability to cope with stress increases your ability to resist illness.

LENT

In Christianity, fasting is a way to cleanse the soul, the body is pure, and it can establish a connection with God. One of the most popular times for Christians to fast is during Lent, which is 40 days from Ash Wednesday to Easter. Once upon a time, those who observed the lent gave up eating and drinking. Nowadays, Christians can still do without food and drink, but often they choose to do without specific things. This practice is said to be a 40-day commendation that Jesus Christ spent in the desert and was forced to fast.

SPIRITUAL FASTING

Fasting was and is an integral part of different religions and spiritual practices around the world. When fasting is used for religious purposes, it is often described as a cleansing or cleansing process, but the basic concept has always been the same: avoid eating for a fixed period.

Unlike medical fasting, which is used to treat illness, spiritual fasting is considered an essential catalyst for the well-being of the whole body, and a variety of religions share the belief that fasting has the power to heal. In Buddhism, fasting is a means of exercising restraint on human desires. A reluctance which, according to Buddhist monks, is part of the puzzle to reach Nirvana. Many Buddhists fast daily, eat in the morning, but abstain for the rest of the day until it is time to eat the next morning. Besides, Buddhists often start fasting with water for days or weeks.

RAMADAN

Ramadan is probably the most famous fasting and an

essential part of the Islamic religion and the ninth month of the Islamic calendar. During Ramadan, Muslims not only stop eating and drinking from dawn until dusk, but also avoid smoking, sexual relationships, and other activities that can be considered guilty. It is believed that periods of fasting and the light dehydration resulting from the lack of body fluids can cleanse the soul from harmful impurities, transform the mind into spirituality and keep it away from worldly desires.

Ramadan is one of the five pillars of Islam.

FIVE INTERMITTENT FASTING VARIANTS

WARRIOR DIET 18-20 HOURS FAST / 4-6 HOURS

This variant is for this reason. It is very intense if you fast in the first 18 to 20 hours of the day or take a particularly recommended meal in combination with your workout. Then consume most of the food within 4-6 hours and then repeat the relining or fasting period. It may be more convenient to place a feeding window at the end of the day. You can adapt it to your schedule at any time.

FAST FOR 36 HOURS EVERY OTHER DAY / 12 HOURS

Feed with this strategy. You eat every other day. It may seem extreme, but the faster, the more experienced, the less worrying you can go about this task. On regular days we only eat 12 hours, for example from 9 a.m. to 9 p.m. Then quickly overnight and quickly 24 hours the next day. Eat the next day again from 9 a.m. to 9 p.m. and fast for a total of 36 hours. In general, everyone can eat faster, which is what they like on days without fasting. However, choosing the right diet leads to better results.

EAT STOP EAT 24 HOURS QUICKLY, 1-2 TIMES A WEEK

This method fasts the entire 24 hours once a week or twice as needed. Then follow a smart diet for the rest of the week. This method is very adjustable. The 24-hour Lent can be any day of your choice.

SKIPPING MEAL

It is a somewhat random approach to fasting. It is a more natural, prehistoric form of fasting. It is believed that our ancestors were not as interested and attached to food as they are today. Nutrition and exercise are random and eat raw healthy food. This method allows you to skip meals 1-2 times a week at random. It is very flexible and no worries.

5: 2 fasting, 5: 2 diet (also known as the 5/2 diet) is a fasting diet plan that limits caloric intake for two days and then eats a regular diet for five days. The general idea behind a 5: 2 diet is to reduce calories for two (non-continuous) days. However, you can eat very low-calorie (but very nutritious) foods two out of seven days a week and the regular diet for the other five days.

LEAN GAINS 16H FAST / 8H FEED - THIS IS THE FAST WE RECOMMEND IN OUR WORKSHOPS

This type of fasting feeds for 8 hours, then 16 hours, but there are additional rules that must be followed. Foods should be high in protein, and carbohydrate intake should be maintained by circulating carbohydrates, such as in an empty stomach or timing nutrition. Training should begin shortly before the end of the 16-hour fast. After exercise, eat the largest of a couple of meals. The fast start again in the evening before bedtime lasts 16 hours and repeats daily. (Be careful! This fast-recommended protocol is for people who are moderately active or above. If you have low sports activity or are new to sports, keep your protein intake low and your carbohydrate intake to a minimum level. Keep in mind, especially simple carbohydrates, which are intended to consume more natural foods and fiber if possible).

Carbohydrates are found in almost all organisms and play an essential role in the proper functioning of the immune system, fertilization, blood coagulation, and human development. Lack of carbohydrates can cause malfunctions in all of these systems. However, the deficiency is rare in the western world. Excessive intake of carbohydrates, incredibly refined carbohydrates such as sugar and corn syrup, can lead to obesity, type II diabetes, and cancer. Unhealthy carbohydrate foods include dried fruits, cereals, crackers, cakes, flours, jams, bread products, and potato products. Healthy carbohydrate foods are vegetables, legumes (beans), whole grains, fruits, nuts, and yogurts.

Fasting has physical and psychological benefits. One of the main advantages of fasting and one of the main reasons why many people fast at times is fat loss. Understanding the difference between a fed and a fasted state can help you know how it works.

The fed state is the state in which our bodies digest and ingest food. It starts with eating and takes 3-5 hours as your body digests and intakes this food. High insulin levels make it challenging to burn fed fat. After digestion and absorption, your body stops processing food. This relaxed mode lasts about 8-12 hours after your last meal, and you are hungry.

In this state, your insulin level is so low that your body is more likely to burn fat. Because of these 12 hours, our body is in a quieter state than when burning fat. Fasting can lead you to this fat-burning condition. It is the number of people who start fasting, burning fat without changing their diet or exercising.

Further advantages have been demonstrated in both animal and animal experiments. Some of these benefits include, but are not limited to, low blood lipids, blood pressure, inflammation markers, oxidative stress, and cancer risk. It also increases cell turnover and repair, fat burning, beneficial growth hormone release, and metabolic rate, as well as the release of other harmful body aging hormones (IGF-1). Finally, the effects of appetite control, blood sugar control, cardiovascular function, chemotherapy, neurogenesis, and neuroplasticity were improved.

Training the mind is the most outstanding achievement of fasting. Psychologically retrain the brain and body's response to hunger. Through fasting, we find that need is not an emergency. Our bodies are trained on how to approach panic and how to curb the desire for immediate satisfaction. It is a great skill you need to master today in the time of the fast-paced modern world. You can see that feeling of hunger is just a feeling. If you are devoted to fasting all day long, you will soon realize that hunger is not upsetting. If you miss a meal, your body will die without switching off. Our prehistoric ancestors did not have fast-food restaurants in every corner. There is a difference between physiological and psychological hunger, and we often confuse the two. Understanding the difference between the two helps you understand the signals in your body. If you feel starving, a record that sensation, usually at the end of a fast, and use it as a reference when you think you are hungry. If you compare the two, you can see which one is hungry.

Eating is a privilege and responsibility that we often receive when we take it for granted. Fasting helps us reassess why we eat and what we incorporate into our bodies. It enables us to recognize that we have little or no food to eat, and we eat our meals every day as usual. Eating processed nutrients without food is also bad for our body, and we are forced to use the feeding window in a more limited and nutritious way. We are always surrounded by endless marketing campaigns targeting consumers. Food ads, especially junk food ads, send subliminal signals that usually fly under the radar when we are full. We store this information and pull it out when we feel hungry. As you fast, you become more aware of the urges, desires, and ways in which these messages need to be fulfilled. The more clearly you see the operation, the less likely you are to lie. Power and control are closely related to consciousness.

Before going into the details of creating a fasting plan, we must first decide why we want to fast. What is its goal? Your diet and exercise program will depend on the goals you are trying to achieve. Next, you need to identify the diet and exercise plan to include based on your goals. How many calories do you eat during your feeding period? How often and for how long do you exercise each week? These are the questions you need to answer before you start fasting. Knowing the answers to these questions will help you succeed in fasting. Pre-programming these items eliminate the additional stress and worry that can arise during planning. There are many websites with tools to calculate calorie intake based on your lifestyle and exercise plans that will help you reach your goals.

When you are ready to plan your diet and workout, the best place to start lifestyle changes is with the exam. It will help determine tolerance and abstinence on an empty stomach. If you are not familiar with fasting, you will notice slight discomfort when starting a fast. It is mainly after a while, as we usually do not refuse our body food. Your body signals to let you know that you are hungry. It is natural, and the stimuli for mood swings and changes in hormone levels are also natural, but when you learn, the meaning of that feeling in the body is the sense of fat loss that begins with others. It can be converted to many benefits. The test should be comfortable and straightforward. Try it for 14-16 hours without a meal. It allows you to feel a deliberate hunger to get used to this feeling. Controlling appetite is essential for weight loss and health. A quick test is also a great way to see if a form of long-term fasting is right for you. Monitor and record the response of your body to this deliberate hunger. You may not want to try to fast for long periods if your reaction is severe and you experience signs of depression, or if you have extreme mood swings or irritation. Try Fast Eat - Pick a day when you do not eat for 14-16 hours on weekdays and do not eat anything.

Here are some things to remember and relieve stress.

- You can have tea and coffee during the fasting period. If you cannot drink it without milk, you can just apply the color with splashes. No sugar is allowed, but artificial sweeteners are acceptable and preferably all-natural stevia.

- During this period, non-calorie soft drinks, chewing gum, and mint are also allowed.
- Drinking water will reduce your hunger. (Hunger is the feeling that the body is burning fat, releasing beneficial growth hormones and repairing cells while lowering the body's release of aging hormones).
- Watch for body signals. If you feel stressed or frustrated during the fast, relax.
- Homes always have healthy food options and are ready to fast. Having healthy food options ensures that there is no temptation to spoil at the end of the fasting period.

Once you have a better understanding of what you expect from a daily fast and you decide that this quick option is what you can take, you are ready to start the lean gains. Eating for 8 hours and then fasting for 16 hours is always "difficult," but "easy." If you can, give yourself time to relax and meditate. It helps you stay focused and remember your goals. I want to make sure your mind and body are in balance.

If you do the math, you can say to yourself, "Are you sure you want to skip breakfast?" The answer is yes, and no! Of course, this is a very controversial approach in today's society. We often hear that breakfast is the most important meal of the day, which is true. However, if you are fasting because you think breakfast is what you meant, you do not have to worry about it every time you eat. Your main concern is to eat healthy when you are fasting. If you have to eat breakfast early in the morning due to your busy schedule or medical reasons, you can schedule a fast this way. Eat your last meal 8 hours before bedtime (assuming you sleep 8 hours). It allows you to exercise and then eat the biggest meal of the day in the morning. It is not the usual planning approach; it has more challenges, but it sometimes works.

Another critical point to remember is that the 16/8 speed is for those who want to be skinny. Having previous fitness and health routine makes this easy. It also seems more comfortable and works better for men. Women can quickly correct this, if necessary, by eating more and reducing hunger. It is especially true if you are generally a busy person and misses the opportunity to eat. If you do not have the time, you may want to increase your meal window to eat healthier. Listen to body signals, especially when you are in the feeding zone. Now you know when to eat, how much to eat and when to eat. Exercises and plans are defined. You can use intermittent fasting to achieve your goals or use it as a permanent lifestyle change, but always pay attention to your body and know what works best for you. Now let us summarize instead of eating several times a day to eat.

SO, WHAT ARE THE STEPS?

1. DETERMINE THE START DATE

We strongly recommend starting on Monday. It makes more sense. After you have selected a day, you can thoroughly prepare for the start time with a few steps.

2. SELECT THE DISTRIBUTION OF FAST / MEAL DETERMINE WHEN TO EAT AND FAST

16/8 is recommended for beginners. You have to get used to it a lot, and it is not too difficult the first time. Select a window and decide when to stop eating the night before fasting. It will serve as a separate house. We recommend that you stick to it for the first week. After practicing FI for a few weeks, it is only natural to change windows and schedules. However, it is best to keep the same time during the first week. So, if you stop eating at 9 p.m. on Sunday, you won't eat at 1 p.m. on Monday. From 1 p.m. to 9 p.m., it will be a dining room window.

3. SPEND A FLIRT DAY

Spend one day on the day before the first fast. Eat a lot and eat whatever you like. It has two purposes. First, the more foods there are in the system, the easier it is to make fast-first. Secondly, if you eat the things you want the night before, that means you won't thirst for these foods for a week.

4. TEACH PEOPLE

I highly recommend talking to your loved ones about the new habits you are adopting. Explain why you do it and why you are hired-politely informed them that you do not eat at certain times and that you will like their support, please. Warn people to make up for your chances of getting food during a fast. One of the most difficult challenges you face is that of a friend, family, or colleague who provides you with food-inform your FI and avoids it.

5. BUY BRANCHED-CHAIN AMINO ACIDS (OPTIONAL)

Branched-chain amino acids (BCAA) are beneficial on an empty stomach. These are pure forms of protein and incredibly powerful for more prolonged fasting. Consuming 10 g of BCAAs can help reduce hunger without fasting. Do not exceed 10 g per serving, but two servings are sufficient during fasting. If you want to exercise, I recommend BCAA.

If you are going to exercise, we recommend that you exercise 60 minutes before and during exercise at one of the following times:

6. TRAINING AND INTERMITTENT FASTING

You do not have to exercise to take advantage of intermittent fasting. However, when you select training, you'll see unprecedented levels of results. As explained earlier in this book, IF increases growth hormone and testosterone production and attacks adipocytes and stores. With the addition of an exercise routine (we recommend strength training), the results you see are incredible. Strength training combined with increased hormones can help you build muscle faster than expected. Lifting weights also increases the production of testosterone and growth hormone, so your body receives twice the dose of hormone production. Weight training is also very metabolic, so shred fat from your body and remember, as I said, you have more muscles, which means less fat.

I would also like to mention that strength training and exercise are probably the most effective way to protect your body from whatever the world throws at you. It has been proven to reduce stress, help with depression, increase energy levels, improve mental function, increase your happiness, improve your life, and help you live longer. Therefore, it is highly recommended to start training. If you do not have a good gym, strength exercises like pushups, squats, and lunges can help you on your journey. Finally, I would like to add one thing, if it can be speeded up, run it. I understand that planning does not mean everyone can do it, but one way to improve is to exercise and fast with a meal after exercise. Do not eat more than 2 hours after weight training, as your muscles will be disrupted, and this will negatively affect your goals.

CHAPTER 5:

THE PROVOCATION OF INTERMITTENT FASTING

If you do this and have spent the first week, you will probably stick to the intermittent fasting lifestyle. The hardest part of fasting is the state of mind we bring to the table. You are not the only one. Millions of people come to

the table with everything but lack nutrition. They come to a family reunion at the table. They comefor the pleasure of the taste and decoration of the food. Theycome from habit, but they do not recognize it. They come to fulfill their obligation to eat even when they are not hungry.

The most important thing when you get to the table is that you think you are going to come there to eat. Consider food to refuel and repair your body. It may be one of the most boring ways of looking at it, but that is precisely what you do. It is time to experience a food revolution and stop thinking about food as a source of pleasure and food as a source of life. Food is part of the life cycle, and food allows us to go out into the world to be more than we currently think about.

BE CAREFUL AND EAT

At the heart of intermittent fasting is a concept that most people only notice when eating when we understand our condition. When it is time to eat, we are usually in a hurry or busy doing other things. It is both a source of entertainment and a source of joy. None of this contributes to a healthy diet.

If you practice intermittent fasting, you need to change your view of the diet and practice a conscious diet.

Conscientious eating is not just about filling, but also about your food and your focus on the food processor. If you eat only twice a day, once in the morning and the afternoon, you should not eat for more than 20 to 30 minutes. Do it quietly and record the experience.

MENTAL FRAMEWORK

Once you have your first experience of intermittent fasting and become familiar with it, you should start clearing your mind. We do this with mindfulness through breathing exercises. Wait, what could you say? What does mind cleaning have to do with intermittent fasting? These are lifestyle changes. Eating how your body is supposed to eat is only part of the equation. For this reason, we then consider some mindfulness practices that I found useful in connection with fasting.

In the first phase, the exercise, you will be introduced to a series of breath and mindfulness exercises. There are four stages you will experience before you realize the effect that will amaze you.

Starting, Stage 1 is easy. Find a comfortable place. There are no other tasks to do with your eyes closed. All you must do is watch your body breathes. If you do this with your eyes closed, it looks like you are looking right above the bridge of your nose, in the middle of your forehead, between your eyes. Identify this as your inner seat.

Watch your breathing as soon as you close your eyes. That is all you have to do. Remember to put on hold all other distractions. When sitting and observing breathing, count the time it takes to inhale until the breath reaches the end of the natural cycle and prepares for expiration.

Remember, you are controlling, not just watching. Whatever respiratory rhythm is part of you right now is what you are looking at. Do not inhale profoundly or change to exhale completely.

LEVEL 1 BREATHE NATURALLY

If you do this, you will know the number of seconds it takes to inhale. Then count the time it takes to exhale. The time it takes to exhale may be the same time it takes to inhale, but it does not matter at this time. All you need to do is to know the number. Do this for the first 10 minutes. As it progresses, expiration can be prolonged compared to inhalation, and breathing can be extended to 15-20 minutes. In the end, open your eyes and relax in the same position, allowing the rest of your life to enter the conscious observation slowly. Listen to each sound as it enters your consciousness. Then open your eyes and let the information overflow.

If you notice the surroundings, remember what you need to remember. What you have seen is that when information is inundated, your mind can only pay attention to one thing.

Repeating this for a week each day will do two things. To slow down and remove all the stress you face, even if you do not know it. But this is only the first part. To understand nature, slowing down is a significant element of success.

HAVE FUN

Fun is not sinful. There are many things you can do in life, but you should not think of all these things for joy. Driving to work every day, paying attention to your car and other drivers on the road, is a conscious experience. Pay attention to driving and routes to your destination. But just because you love racing cars on weekends does not mean you have to drive fast on the road. Eating is eating. Enjoying means entertainment. Eating can be fun, but it is an exception and not standard.

The power of intermittent fasting is to distract the focus and habits of unnatural and unhealthy things. It removes your body's dependence on repeated food intake and deprives it of where it belongs, the resources it is stored on. It also controls the type of food and increases your dependence on a healthy appetite. The power of intermittent fasting is that it is a liberalizing promise that allows you to take control of your life.

JUNK FOOD

The exception to the grocery list is processed junk food. This term is used in this book without exaggeration. Junk food is undesirable for your health and changes your taste from healthy to its reciprocal.

Why choose a healthy diet and continue to avoid processed foods? You can eat s**t and lose weight during an intermittent fast. It is not a permanent solution. You will lose the excess fat, but your body will eventually break down. Be careful what you put in your mouth.

LEVEL 2 CONTROLLED BREATHING

The second part is when you start to control your breathing so that it corresponds to the hours of inspiration and progress. By adjusting the times, you intentionally control your breathing. But do not skip this step right away. You must take it slow. You probably look like 99% of the people in the world, and your breathing techniques are wrong. If you learned to breathe at a young age, your diaphragm is muscular, and you can control your pace well.

As you practice this breathing technique, you will notice that, apart from the best breathing habits and the silence of your mind, your extremities start to tingle. It just means that your pulse oxygen rate is increasing. You send more oxygen to the rest of your body, and it wakes up. With this simple exercise, with little effort, you began to cleanse your body and oxidize most of the gaseous toxins present. Faster weekly water also cleans the colon and improves blood quality. As blood quality improves and breathing increases, enough oxygen flows, and cells are activated. Increasing vitamin C in the fruits, you are currently eating as an alternative to junk food also helps the immune system improve its performance.

LEVEL 3 VISUALIZE DISTRACTIONS

The third stage of meditation helps to end eating habits and pave the way for good health. The third step is pretty easy too. You just need to increase the time you spend on meditation.

The idea is to visualize your pastime, and the food is a

pastime. When we reach this stage, we recognize that we are distracted but not distracted. You will find that your thoughts have their mind. These thoughts are beyond you and separate you from the random pieces of view. Do not worry - everyone has it.

If you watch your breath, you will find that you can monitor everything that is going on around you. When I looked at the same thing, I started to understand not only what I was doing with my breath, but also what I was doing in my heart. You can see the ideas that have become more visible in the eyes of your mind without interacting with them.

The advantage of this third step is that you become the master of the mind. Therefore, it can reduce stress in many situations. To enjoy the benefits, never stop daily meditation routines and weekly fasting.

Just as fasting and vegetarianism cleanse the body, mindfulness and breathing exercises cleanse the mind.

The mindfulness exercises you practice can remind you of an outstanding truth: past and future are not necessary, but moments are essential. Mindfulness is at this moment. When you try to do something in this world, the vital thing in the world is to be in this moment.

LEVEL 4 INSTANT FOCUSES

When you reach this stage, the idea is to control your breathing instantly, which is, what your heart is doing instantaneously, your current position. And, if possible, you have reached the height of simple meditation—no need to visualize anything. Your breath is the strongest in the world.

Between your heart and your breath, there is very little you cannot heal. In Stage 4, it is time to move meditation to other parts of life. Pay attention to what you do everywhere.

Make sure you are at the moment, wherever you are, especially when you are eating. Be careful whether you are on the bus or an airplane. Being mindful does not mean being withdrawn. You are fully aware of what is happening around you. You do not participate, but you see.

There are ups and downs, like everything in life, you experience intermittent fasting, mostly ups and downs at the beginning. Do not expect everything to go smoothly from the start or be wholly absorbed in it.

CHAPTER 6:

WHEN WILL YOU START?

If you do not have a fundamental health problem and you are not a fasting individual, you do not have this time. Ask yourself: When is it not now? It is advisable to wait for the advice of your doctor. You can choose to prepare, get rid of eating habits that are too long, empty the refrigerator, eat the last cookie in a jar, or scratch yourself. Or you may want to continue after a few weeks to see any visible progress. But let's start with the day when you feel healthy, decisive, calm, and committed. Tell your friends and family that you are about to start a fast diet. If you make a public promise, you are more likely to stick to it. Avoid busy days, holidays, days of three-course lunches that include bread baskets, cheeseboards, and four desserts. Also, busy days can help reduce flight times, while quilt days usually crawl like honey with a spoon. When you think about the beginning of the day and specify it, you'll be moved. Before you start, record your details such as weight, BMI, and goals, and record your progress in the journal. Dieters are more likely to losepounds if they honestly record what they eat and drink. Keepthem and take a deep breath and relax.

Better shrug yourshoulders. It does not matter as you lose nothing but weight. How tough will it be? If you've been hungry for a while andeven with a few pointers, eating at least 500 or 600 calories a day, at least initially, can prove to be an easy challenge. Intermittent fasters report that the process becomes much easier over time. Mainly because the results are obtained with mirroring and scaling. The first early days are accelerating, supported by the novelty of the process. The early days of the third week of wet Wednesday may feel like a slogan. Your mission is to complete it. You say no to chocolate today, but tomorrow you will eat whatever you want. This is the joy of a fast diet and a big difference to other weight loss plans. How to win a hunger game!

There is no reason to be surprised by benignity, and occasionally, short-term hunger. If you are in good health, it will not be destroyed. They do not collapse in a heap and need to be saved by the cat. Your body is designed to be food-free for long periods, even if you lose your ability due to years of grazing, hunting, and snacking. Studies show that modern people tend to confuse different emotions with hunger. When I'm bored, thirsty, when I'm near food (when it is not), when they're together or when the clock tells us it is time to eat. Most of us also eat because we feel good. This is known as "hedonic hunger." You should try to resist the fasting days, but you can rely on your knowledge to lose the temptation the next day if necessary. You do not have to panic about it. Note that the human brain is good at persuading us to be hungry in almost any situation. You are faced with deprivation, withdrawal, or disappointment when you are angry, sad, happy, or neutral. The smell of freshly brewed coffee in a roadside cafe when influenced by advertising, social demands, sensory stimuli, rewards, and habits. Realize now that these are often learned reactions to external cues, and most of them are designed to let you get out of your money.

If you are still preparing your last meal, it is unlikely that you will feel starving ("total transit time" if you are interested in things like sex, metabolism, and what you ate). Hunger can be as aggressive and uncomfortable as a sharp knife box, but it is more fluid and controllable than you might imagine. I'm not even hungry before the day of fasting begins. Also, the blow passes. Fasters report that the perception of hunger is riding the waves and not the walls of the ever-growing stomach bite. It is a symphony of differentiated movements, not a horrifying and endless crescendo. Treat the belly rumble as a good sign, a healthy messenger.

Also, do not always feel hungry, as you will not feel hungry for more than 24 hours. Wait a minute. You have the absolute power to overcome the feelings of hunger, just by turning your mind, riding the waves and doing other things- walking, calling friends, drinking tea, running, take a shower, take a shower and sing, get a friend from the rain and sing. It is commonly reported that after a few weeks of intermittent fasting, my hunger decreased. As we have seen, one of the most critical studies examining how obese people respond to intermittent fasting is the more sophisticated Alternative Day-Modified Fasting Method (ADMF) at the University of Chicago. Volunteers did it. In this study, "we found that hunger levels increased and corrected hunger every other day for the first week. However, after two weeks of ADMF, hunger levels decreased and remained low throughout the rest of the study." "This indicates that the subject is accustomed to the ADMF diet after about two weeks (that is, they are not very hungry on a fasting day)." "The ADMF diet was less satisfied in the first four weeks of the intervention, but gradually increased in the last four weeks of the study."

In short, researchers suggest that obese participants may be able to continue their diet over a more extended period as their feeling of hunger decreases significantly, and their satisfaction with their diet improves considerably in the short term. I decided it was high. The study was conducted with people who fasted every other day. In contrast, partial fasting two days a week - a fast diet plan - is discouraging. Take courage. Avoid, restrain, distract, fast. Before you know it, you are retraining your brain and starving from the menu. Tomorrow is another day: delayed strength, patience, and satisfaction.

Perhaps the safest and most innovative part of a fast diet is that it does not last forever. Unlike the lousy food that had failed before, this plan will always be different tomorrow. Simpler breakfast, including pancakes, lunch with friends, and wine, cream, and apple pies for dinner. This on / off switch is essential. So, on fasting days, you eat a quarter of your regular calorie intake, but tomorrow you can eat as much as you want. The fact that a fast is a short stay and a short break after a meal offers endless psychological comfort.

Unlike a full-time fad diet, you still enjoy food, you will always have a snack, and you will attend regular and routine eating events in your everyday life. No special shakes, bars, rules, points, ailments, or singularities. However, do not always say "no." You ought to not feel like you've been robbed immediately. Like all those who have embarked on the tedious task of a long-term daily diet, the kind of persons who want to execute the Hara-kiri on the kitchen floor.

Traditional meal plans fail when you open the refrigerator door. The key is to recognize that breakfast can be reached through the exercise of patience and willpower. The flavor sings—stab dance. If you have, without thinking, felt lazy disdain for the food you eat, then things are about to change. There is nothing like the satisfaction that has been postponed. A bit to make things better—compliance and sustainable: how to find smart meal models that work for you??

Most diets do not work. You already know it. Indeed, when a team of UCLA psychologists performed an analysis of 31 long-term diet trials in 2007, their analysis found that skinny people had lost pounds in the first few months, while the majority will return to their original weight in a year. Conclusively, the researchers agreed that most of the participants would have better been off not going for the diet plans at all. Losing the weight and gaining it back made their bodies to suffer wear and tear. Another massive study on a group of 19000 older people with two categories: people with diet history before the conduct of the study and people with no diet history. For four years, it was observed that people with no diet history were better off than the others in the group.

Therefore, to be effective, each method must be rational, sustainable, flexible, and long-term viable. What matters is not adherence to weight loss, but adherence itself. Therefore, the objectives must be realistic, and the program should be practical. It should fit into your life, not the life of your dreams but where you live. Any weight loss strategy must be tolerable, organic, and innate. It is not a fake supplement equivalent to a food resembling a good looking but an unpleasant shoe.

LONG TERM EXPERIENCE

The long-term experience of intermittent fasting is still being researched, but those who have tried it commented, how easily it fits into everyday life. They always get food variety (anyone who has tried to lose weight with the "only" grapefruit or cabbage soup knows how important it is). They always get rewards from food. They still have a life; there is no drama, no hopeless system, no masturbation. Do not sweat.

FLEXIBILITY: THE KEY TO SUCCESS

Your body is not my body. Mine is not yours. It is, therefore, worthwhile to adapt your plan to your needs, your day form, your family, your commitment, and your taste. None of us live a cookie-cutter, and a diet is not for everyone. Everyone has habits and modifiers. Therefore, there is no absolute command here, only suggestions. You can choose to fast in a certain way on a particular day and also first or last one or two times.

Some people want to know precisely what and when to eat. Others prefer a more informal approach. It is nice just to follow the primary method (500 calories or 600 calories twice a day, long without meals) twice a week, and you will reap the many benefits of the plan. Ultimately, you rarely need to do a dedicated calorie count. You know what a fast day means and how you can adapt it to your needs.

MAINTENANCE MODEL

You can consider a maintenance model as soon as you reach your target weight or shadow below it (providing range and abundant birthday cakes). It adjusts to fasting only once a week to maintain a maintenance pattern at the desired weight, but still utilizes fasting occasionally. Of course, if you wish, one day a week will give you fewer health benefits than two days in the long run. But it fits perfectly in life, especially if you are not going to achieve further weight loss.

What to expect: the first thing you can expect when dieting fast is to lose weight. In some weeks, you will find yourself stuck in a disappointing plateau, and in others, you will progress more quickly. As an essential guide, you could expect to lose around a pound per day of fasting. Of course, it is not all bold. However, you will need to lose about 10 pounds of fat in 10 weeks compared to an everyday low-calorie diet. The key is to maintain weight loss over time.

HOW YOUR ANATOMY CHANGES?

BMI, body fat levels and waist size are expected to decrease gradually over the next few weeks. It should also improve your cholesterol and triglyceride levels. It is the path to better health and longer life. You are already dodging your unwritten future. But for now, as your body becomes thinner and lighter, noticeable changes begin to appear in the mirror.

For several weeks, you can see that intermittent fasting also has significant side effects. In addition to noticeable weight loss and preserved health benefits for the future, more subtle results, benefits and bonuses, may work. Changes in appetite expect your eating preferences to adjust. From now on, we opt for healthy food as standard and not for design. They start to understand, negotiate, and deal with hunger, and to know what it feels like to be hungry.

Instead of moaning like an immobile sofa, you can also see a feeling of comfort and fullness. I am full and not a filling. What is the result? "Food hangover," improved digestion, no crack.

Interesting eating habits appear six months after a temporary fast. You may be eating half of the meat you eat once, not as a conscious movement, but as a natural movement that comes from what you want, rather than making a decision or believing. You can consume more vegetables. Many intermittent fasters instinctively withdraw from bread (and in some cases, butter), strange "comfort" foods are less attractive, and refined sugar is less attractive than before.

Hairdo's bag in the glove compartment of the car? Take it or leave it. Of course, you do not have to be proactive. It happens anyway. If you are a person like me, you'll someday arrive at a place you hate cheesecake. Not because I hate it, but because I refuse to treat myself. This is the raw power of intermittent fasting: it encourages you to check your diet. And this is your long-distance health ticket how your attitude changes.

So yes, you will start losing the bad eating habits. However, if you continue to notice and continue to fast and treat, all other types of changes should occur.

For example, you may suffer from "partial distortion" for years because you think the dishes on the plate are needed and needed. Over time, you will find that you are overdoing it. The muffin sits under the glass dome of the coffee shop, and when it is thick and moist, it looks big. The potato chips maxi bag makes an expansive view. To get from Venti to Grande, you only need half a cup, no sugar, no cream. You will soon become aware of what you have eaten and what unspoken wording you have been saying for years. The progression of doing so is more than anything else as part of the readjustment process.

I've changed my mind. Occasionally, fasting trains you in the art of "restricted nutrition." In the last example, this is the goal. It is all part of a long-acting game, which means that the fast diet ultimately does not become a fast diet, but a way of life.

After a while, you will develop a new approach to dietary, rational, and responsible eating, even if you do not even know you are. Intermittent fasting also reports increased energy and increased emotional well-being. Some people talk about "shine." Perhaps the result of winning a struggle for self-control or something that happens in smaller clothes, compliments, or at the metabolic level that determines our mood. I still do not know the exact reason, but I feel good. Much better than a cake.

Online fans say: "Overall, fasting seems right. It is like a reset button for your whole body." Even more subtly, I feel reassured as many fasts are no longer eating on their fasting days. Accept it. If you allow it, you have some freedom here. You may find that we look forward to fasting as we do.

FEMALE SPEED: MIMI'S EXPERIENCE

Most men I know respond well to numbers and goals

(preferably using related gadgets), but I have found that women tend to take a more comprehensive approach to fast. Knowing that our body is unique and responds to stimuli given in its way, like many things in life, we want to find out what it does. Respond to shared stories and support from friends. And sometimes a snack is needed.

Personally, for example, I burn fasting calories in two batches, one fast and one late, to spare a day to limit and maximize profit prospects. Aim for a longer gap between the two: Health and weight loss. But in the meantime, I need a little something to keep me. A simple breakfast is usually low sugar muesli, probably containing strawberries, fresh almonds, and semi-skimmed milk. Then dinner: lots of leaves and lean protein-probably smoked salmon, tuna, or hummus-when a child goes into bed, a substantial and exciting salad. All-day long, I drink San Pellegrino mineral water with a splash of lime, lots of herbal tea, and lots of black coffee. They just help the day go by. In the four months since the fast diet started, I have lost 6 kg, and my BMI has changed from 21.4 to 19.4. If you are struggling with larger numbers, take advantage of the fact that more obese subjects respond wonderfully to intermittent fasting. The positive effects can be seen in a relatively short time. Nowadays, weekly fasting (Monday) is enough and seems to hold a stable and happy weight.

Many of the women I meet are familiar with diet techniques (longstanding practice), and I have found a few tips to help on a short day. For example, we recommend eating with a small bite, chewing slowly, and concentrating while eating. Why do you read magazines, and why do you mumble while eating? If you only get 500 calories, it makes sense to notice this while taking it.

Hunger turned out to be more than just a problem like many occasionally accelerated cases. For some reason - and we're wondering if it is suitable for the food industry - we've been plagued by fear of hunger, hypoglycemia, and more. On the whole, days with less food are more liberal than limiting me. It means that there are ups and downs: for a few days, it will fly like stones on water. On other days, I feel like I'm sinking and not swimming. Probably because emotions, hormones, or the tricky business of life has started. See how you feel and always give grace when this is special.

6 WAYS TO MAKE A FAST DIET EFFECTIVE

1. KNOW YOUR WEIGHT, BMI AND WAIST SIZE FROMTHE START

As mentioned earlier, the waist measurement is an essential and straightforward measure of internal fat and a strong predictor of future health. People with intermittent fasting quickly lose those dangerous and unattractive centimeters. The BMI is the square of the weight (in kilograms) divided by the height (in meters). It looks ugly and may sound abstract, but it is a widely used tool to find a way to healthy weight loss. The BMI values do not take into account your body type, age, or ethnicity. You should, therefore, greet them informed. However, this is useful when you need a number.

Weigh yourself regularly. After the first phases, once a week is sufficient. If you want the numbers to drop, the morning after fasting is your best bet. Researchers at the University of Illinois noted: "Weighing can vary significantly from food to fasting days. This weight deviation is probably due to the extra weight of food in the digestive tract.

It is not a daily change in fat mass. Future solutions may require solutions that try averaging the weight measurements on consecutive feeding and fasting days to determine weight more accurately. There are 28 tasks. If you are a person who likes structure and clarity, you may want to track your progress. Think about your goals. When and where do you want to go? Be realistic: rapid weight loss is not recommended. Please take your time. Make a plan. Write it down.

Many people recommend keeping a diet journal. Add your experience next to the number. Note the three good things that happen every day. It is a message of happiness that can be referenced over time.

2. FIND A QUICK FRIEND

You need very few accessories to be successful, but a supportive friend can be one of them. Once you are on the fast diet, tell people about it; You may find that they join you, and you will build a network of shared experiences. As the plan appeals to both men and women, couples report that doing it together is more comfortable. This way, you get mutual support, camaraderie, shared engagement, and shared anecdotes. Also, mealtimes are infinitely more comfortable if you eat with someone who understands the basics of the plot.

There are also many discussions in online discussion forums. Mums net are an excellent source of support and information. It is remarkable how reassuring it is to know that you are not alone.

3. QUICK MEAL PREPARATION

Prepare your quick meal in advance, so you do not have to search for food and come across a sausage that irresistibly hides in the fridge. Keep it simple and effortlessly strive for the taste of the day. Buy and cook on non-fast days to avoid laughing at inappropriate temptations. Clean the house of junk food before embarking. It will only sing and coo in the closets, making your fasting day more difficult than it should be.

4. CHECK THE PARTIAL SIZE OF THE CALORIE LABEL

If the serial box says "30 g", weigh it. Continue. Be surprised. Then be honest. Your calorie count is necessarily fixed and limited on an empty stomach, so it is important not to worry about how much is flowing. Here, you'll find our recommended fast food calorie counters. More importantly, do not count calories on the late days.

You have better things. Wait before you eat. Resist at least 10 minutes, and preferably 15 minutes, to see if your hunger subsides (which is usually the case). If you need a snack, choose one that does not raise your insulin levels. Try carrot carrots, a handful of popcorn, apple slices, or strawberries. But do not pinch like chicken all day. Calories are stacked up quickly, and your fasting is fast. Eat consciously on a fasting day and fully absorb the fact that you are eating (especially if you have ever been in a massive traffic jam). Also, be careful with your vacation. Do not eat until you are satisfied (of course, this happens after a few weeks of practice). Find out what the concept of "satisfaction" means to you. We are all different, and it changes over time.

5. STAY BUSY

"We humans are always looking for activities between meals," Leonard Cohen said. Yes, see where it takes us. So, fill your day, not your face. "No one is hungry during the first few seconds of skydiving," said Brad Pilon, the advocate of fasting. Distraction is the best defense against the dark art of the food industry, with doughnuts and nachos on every corner. If you need this doughnut, keep in mind that it will remain tomorrow.

6. TRY 2 TO 2

Fast from 2:00 p.m. to 2:00 p.m., not from bedtime to bedtime. After lunch on the first day, eat modestly until late lunch on the next day.

This way, you will lose weight during sleep and will not feel uncomfortable for a day without food. This is a smart trick, but it requires a bit more focus than the all-day option. Alternatively, you can go from dinner to dinner quickly. In short, no day is fast and fun. The point is that this plan is "adapted to adjustment." Just like your waistband in 3 weeks.

A TERRIBLE FAST FOR WOMEN?

Women's bodies are designed to carry babies physiologically, making them more susceptible to starvation than men. When a woman's body detects impending famine, it responds by increasing the hormones leptin and ghrelin that work together to control appetite. This hormonal response is the means the female body uses to protect the developing fetus, even if the woman is not currently pregnant.

It is possible to ignore the hunger signals of ghrelin and lepton, but this becomes increasingly difficult, mainly as the body repels and begins to produce more of these hormones. If a woman becomes hungry in an unhealthy way-eating too much or eating unhealthy food-this can cause a chain of other hormonal problems related to insulin.

This process can also shut down the reproductive system. If the body believes that there is not enough food to survive, it can affect the ability to conceive to protect the chances of pregnancy. For this reason, fasting is not recommended for women who are pregnant or trying to conceive.

The hypothalamic-pituitary-gonadal axis (HPG) controls the endocrine glands involved in ovulation. The first part of the evaluation process is the release of gonadotropin-releasing hormone (GnRH) from the hypothalamus. The release of GnRH then triggers the pituitary gland and releases both the follicle-stimulating hormone (FSH) and the luteinizing hormone (LH). In women, the release of FSH and LH causes the ovaries and the production of estrogenic and progesterone. Increased estrogenic and progesterone cause the release of mature eggs (ovulation). This hormonal cascade usually occurs in regular cycles. However, GnRH is extremely sensitive and can be discarded by fasting.

This does not mean that intermittent fasting is not appropriate for women. That means you should be a little more careful about it. If you are the first fasting woman and you are trying to see if that's right for you, then you should start a fasting crescendo.

Crescendo fasting only fasts for 12-16 hours a few days a week, not every day. These short days should not be consecutive (e.g., Tuesday, Thursday, Saturday). On fast days, you should only do light exercises such as yoga or walking. Intense activities such as strength training should be booked for a few days without fasting when eating a regular meal. Drinking plenty of water is also essential. A general recommendation is ounces and half weight. Therefore, if you weigh 140 pounds, you should drink at least 70 ounces of water each day. Of course, the amount of water you need depends on many factors, such as your age, weight, activity level, and amount of coffee you drink. However, you should use this equation as a basis.

If you feel good after a few weeks of crescendo fasting, you can add another day fasting and see how your body responds. If you still feel good, you can add more days until you reach your fasting goal. The main point of Crescendo's fasting is to relax slowly and, at the same time, not to over-impact the body. The smaller the plate, the better.

It may be a trick in the head, but the small plates help control the parts. If you have a dish, you tend to fill it up. This means that you usually serve more meals on a large plate than on a small scale. Instead of a dinner plate, choose a salad or starter plate. If you are still hungry, you can always go back a few seconds, but take some time for the food to calm down. In many cases, it is recommended to wait 5-10 minutes between eating and returning to your next help. It gives your body the ability to decide if you are starving.

FASTING AND FUSSING

There is a general belief that if you eat too long, you end up eating unhealthy foods and eventually gain weight. Not so black and white. There are many factors to consider.

Fasting studies every other day show that fasting people tend to eat more calories the day after a 24-hour fast. However, the increase is less than 500 calories. Even if you include the calorie loss on an empty stomach in a minimal rise in next day intake, you are running out of calories.

Often, the desire for bulimia is also caused by a dramatic drop in blood sugar that occurs after a high-carbohydrate meal, or by carbohydrate addiction. As soon as the blood sugar level drops after a period of intermittent fasting, the feeling of hunger stabilizes, and the tendency to overeat decreases.

For people suffering from bulimia and eating disorders, fasting can lead to seizures. If you have had an eating disorder in the past, be sure to consult your doctor before beginning an intermittent fast.

CHOOSE THE RIGHT MEAL

The term "nutrition" is often associated with specific food restrictions. Still, the primary definition of nutrition is "the type of food that a person normally eats," so it is necessary to interpret the term here. Please note that there are no special diets you must follow for intermittent fasting, but choosing a diet with nutritious, unprocessed foods will, of course, be the most effective. Some different diets are popular for intermittent fasting but are not involved in the doctrine. You do not have to follow your diet plan exactly as described. For example, if you choose an old template, but find that your body responds well to brown rice, you can add it. It is not necessary to permanently exclude food just because it does not fall under the title of diet. Use intuitive food to find the best approach.

INGREDIENTS FOR HEALTHY FASTING-FOOD

Intermittent fasting is not just about eating. It will also let you know what you eat. Just as there are different ways to fast, there are other diets you can follow, including old foods, low carbs, and pagans. You need to find one that works for you and achieve what you want. Also, you need to make the right decisions when buying foods to find foods and beverages that promote maximum health.

If you already have a reasonable and happy weight, you can still fast effectively, but you should consider adjusting your intake on non-fast days to get more caloric foods. The leading researchers we spoke to in this area are all skinny and always fast. With practice, you will discover a nice balance between fasting and eating that will keep your weight within the prescribed range. Fast once a week, not twice a week. There are no specific studies to shed light on the effects, but use your common sense and look at the scales.

Do not slide as mentioned above, the fasting of any kind is not recommended if you are already skinny or have an eating disorder. If in doubt, contact your family doctor. How long do you need to continue?

Interestingly, the fast diet on/off diet is very similar to the approach of many naturally lean people. One day they will choose the other day they will treat themselves to a treat. In the long run, this is how fast diet works. Once in the routine, it will naturally adjust its caloric intake on fasting and eating days until the process is natural. Once you reach your target weight, you can change the frequency of fasting. Play with it, but do not drift. Be careful. Your goal is a permanent life change, not a moment, not a trend, not a cat for dinner. It is a long-distance road to sustainable weight loss. Accept to do it in a way that suits you indefinitely as long as you are alive.

FASTING FUTURE: WHERE TO GO FROM HERE?

As I mentioned at the beginning of the book, fasting has been practiced for thousands of years, but science has just caught up. The first evidence of the long-term benefits of calorie reduction was found about 80 years ago. A nutritionist who worked with rats at Cornell University in the US found that they could live longer if their diet was severely restricted.

Since then, there has been growing evidence that animals are calorie-restricted, not only when they live longer and healthier, but also when they starve at times. In recent years, rodent research has shifted to humans, and we see the same pattern of improvement.

So where are you going from here? Professor Valter Longo, who has done many pioneering studies with IGF-1, is working with colleagues at the University of Southern California on several human studies that examine the effects of fasting on cancer. You have already shown that fasting lowers the risk of cancer. Now they want to see whether fasting also improves the effectiveness of chemotherapy and radiation therapy. Dr. Krista Varady of the University of

Illinois at Chicago is planning several projects. Research is currently underway to investigate how long-term people can withstand ADF. This is a critical study because the success or failure of a diet depends entirely on compliance.

Are people still looking forward to it? The last time we talked to each other, she also found out why people with ADF lose fat but not big muscles, and people with ADF do not completely burn the calories you have. He was again talking about future ideas, including research on why they didn't make up for them missed eating more on their feeding day. She has many theories but needs colder and harder facts.

Professor Mark Mattson of the National Institutes of Aging, Baltimore, is continually adding to dozens of previously published studies on the effects of fasting and intermittent fasting on the brain. In particular, I'm particularly keen to see the results of some of his recent studies, including further research into what happens to the minds of volunteers when they undergo intermittent fasting. Also, his team is considering drug therapy. Despite its benefits, it is used, for example, in the treatment of diabetes because it knows that many may not want to fast, but it activates the production of BDNF (the neurotrophic factor from the brain). This seems to protect the brain from aging damage, as we've seen. Even if Vietta or a related drug does not prevent dementia, it at least slows down its progression considerably. Intermittent fasting is one of the best-kept secrets of science.

STARTING INTERMITTENT FASTING YOUR FIRST 30 DAYS

Week 1 – In week one you are simply going to adapt to the window.
Tasks
1. Choose your preferred eight hour eating window. Remember
sleep is allocated to your fasting window. Try to base your eating window within times you feel it will be hardest not to eat and show discipline.
2. Do not change the type of food you eat drastically. This week
is about getting used to the eating window.
3. Do not exercise. If you are new to fasting exercise will most
probably spike hunger making discipline harder. Only focus on
staying within your window.
4. Practice the 16:8 method Monday – Friday and have the weekend off.

Week 2 – If you managed to stick to the tasks outlined in week 1, move on to the tasks set out below. This week we will address sleep, and continue to practice the 16:8 eating pattern.
Tasks
1. Assess last weeks eating window. Do you need to change it? Does it fit with your schedule? If yes, continue to practice this window Monday - Friday. If no, Select a new eating window and repeat week 1.
2. Implement one of the four tips for better sleep outlined earlier in this book from Monday – Friday

3. Feel free to lightly exercise if you have itchy feet! However, I
would still recommend no exercise if you are struggling with hunger to allow full adaptation of your eating window.
4. Again, do not change the type of food you eat drastically.

Week 3 – This week we will add exercise. You've probably been hanging out to burn some calories if you haven't already started!
Tasks
1. Access your eating window. Is it still working? Does it need to
change to help you be more disciplined? If the window is fine
continue with your current window Monday – Friday. If not, select a new window and return to week 1.
2. Add appropriate HITT training based on your ability level. Remember; always consult a relevant professional before under
going any diet or exercise plan.
3. Continue to practice your selected tip for sleep quality from the previous week.
4. Start cutting back sugar.

Week 4 - By week four you should have your ideal eating window in place.
Tasks
1. Continue with your chosen eating window Monday-Friday
2. Add some of the foods outlined under electrolytes for added
magnesium and potassium.

3. Research healthy dessert options to help keep sane! The trick here is to find keto desserts as they will be high in fat and low in
carbohydrates. Remember, fat spikes less insulin and will help
your body switch to using fat for energy. Don't believe the "low
fat" agenda 3 for ideas.
4. Continue to eliminate sugar
5. Perform 2-4 HITT workouts

As you can see, the first 30 days of 16:8 is not drastic. I have not outlined giving up bread, potato or even sweet treats. Your first 30 days should be spent making positive changes, and attaining great results to keep you motivated to continue. The key to long term success lays in how you start.

I advise against rushing forward as a beginner, even though I know how desperate you are for results. The number one reason people give up initially is from trying too much, too soon. Sometimes, we have spent 5 – 20 years being overweight or unhealthy.

It is unreasonable to expect yourself to reverse life long habits and lack of discipline in the blink of an eye!

Tips to Survive IF

Some people can go for 24 hours or more without food but for others, it is a real struggle to go for as little as six hours
There are a few ways to help you cope.

1. **Stay Hydrated** - sometimes our bodies interpret dehydration
as hunger. You may feel those hunger pangs and think, 'Oh I
need to eat something'. Sometimes all you need to do is sip

something. While fasting, take lots of water. You can also drink black coffee, black tea, sparkling water and other zero calorie drinks.

2. **Stay Busy** – Have you ever been hungry at work but not had the chance to eat? Often, when you finally get the chance to eat you're not actually hungry anymore. By staying busy, you can replicate this. Remember hunger comes in waves.

3. **Give It Time** – Sometimes we get too impatient, especially when it comes to losing weight. We diet or exercise for two days then we check the scale and the mirror to see 'the big change' and then we get disappointed. What happens when you get disappointed? You fall off the wagon. If you want to get anywhere with IF, you must give it time. First, allow the eating pattern time to do its wonders to your body. You only need to keep going and the change will show itself.

4. **Give Your Body Time To Adapt To Fasting** - You just stopped eating six meals a day every day. Your body may react differently now that it has to make do with fewer meals.

Hunger, headaches and sometimes body weakness are among the discomforts you may experience. Don't give up! Use logic though. Keep it Safe!

CHAPTER 7:

SHOULD YOU FAST?

Fasting is suitable for most healthy people, but some groups should not fast, and others should speak to their health care team before starting fasting.

Do not fast if:

- If you are pregnant or breastfeeding
- Severe weight loss or malnutrition
- Under 18 years

Talk to your doctor before fasting if you have:

- To take medicine
- History of eating disorders
- Cortisol deregulation or severe stress
- Diabetes (type 1 or 2)
- GERD (Gastroesophageal Reflux Disease)

LISTEN TO YOUR BODY

Listen carefully to your body to see if fasting is right for you. If you experience low energy or dizziness while standing, you may need to adjust your fasting time or consult a doctor to make sure your body can regulate your blood sugar properly. Remember that it takes a long time for your body to get used to your new lifestyle. There is usually a transition period of 3-6 weeks during which your body and brain adapt to hunger. During this time, appetite, irritability, weakness, and even loss of libido occurs. This is a normal response.

However, if your symptoms are severe, call your doctor at these early stages. If you feel good after the conditioning phase, this is a good sign that your body likes your behavior. If, after this, you feel dizzy, lightheaded, or low in energy, stop fasting, and consult a doctor.

FASTING AND DIABETES

Fasting can be a challenge for people with diabetes, as the body has more difficulty controlling their blood sugar and insulin levels than people without diabetes. However, studies have shown that intermittent fasting can help restore normal glucose levels. The main concern with fasting and diabetes is hypoglycemia or hypoglycemia.

GET DOCTOR APPROVAL

If you have diabetes, make sure you have your doctor's approval and supervision before you start your fast. If your doctor has approved intermittent fasting, you should be familiar with the symptoms of hypoglycemia and plan for treatment if your blood sugar becomes too low. If your blood sugar exceeds 300 milligrams per deciliter or falls below 70 milligrams per deciliter, stop hunger immediately, and give appropriate treatment.

MANAGE CHRONIC ILLNESSES

The stress that fasting has on the body can be classified as stress for most people. It offers health benefits that will help you achieve your ultimate goals. However, if you are already experiencing chronic pain, you need to control it before you include intermittent fasting in your routine. With chronic stress, your body continuously excretes cortisol. If cortisol levels remain elevated for an extended time, they can cause:

- Anxiety
- Depression
- Sleepiness
- Digestive problems
- A headache
- Heart disease
- Memory and concentration problems
- Weight gain

Over time, chronic stress can also affect adrenal function, making it challenging to regulate hormones properly. If you are already experiencing chronic stress, it is essential to control cortisol levels and make the adrenal gland function properly before fasting.

Meditation can help lower cortisol levels. Avoid coffee, sleep well, and eat clean and healthy for a while before fasting. Avoid excessive exercise. A yoga-like, low-impact meditation exercise can help.

PREPARE FOR FASTING

Except for spontaneous fasting, most types of intermittent fasting require some preparation. One of the most important things you can do to prepare for your fast is to develop a plan. What kind of intermittent fasting will you do? What days and times will you fast? What is your official start date? It helps to create a schedule for yourself and keep it where you can see it at all times. You can even set your phone's timers to run out when it is time to start fasting and when it is time to start eating again. But you do not have to go straight to a defined fasting plan. You can slowly relax to understand.

STARTING YOGA

In a study by the Yoga Research Society and Sidney Kimmel Medical College at Thomas Jefferson University, the researchers found that after a fifty-minute yoga class, the cortisol levels were decreased. Yoga poses like tree-laying, low-laying, and grasshopper-laying became popular. The researchers believe that this decrease in cortisol is due in part to the activation of the relaxation response by holding poses and breathing deeply. This relaxation reaction reduces the stress cascade, and therefore stress hormones are naturally reduced. High cortisol levels are also expected in people with depression. A study published in the Indian Journal of Psychiatry found that yoga can help 'stop' the stress response in the hypothalamus area of the brain, which can help people with depression. The study found that yoga was more popular than antidepressants.

MAKE FASTING EASY

If you are not accustomed to intermittent fasting, or if you are accustomed to small meals or grazing 5-6 times a day, a straight transition to fasting can be a big transition. You do not have to make a complete change overnight. You'll be more successful if you get used to it slowly.

Start by moving from 5 or 6 small meals to 3 regular size meals throughout the day.

You do not have to eat in a certain amount of time. You

will only get used to the habits and structure of the three-meal schedule.

You also need to get rid of snacks all day long. Snacks are not prohibited if you are occasionally fasting, but you can adjust by eliminating early snacks. Once you get used to fasting, you can eat snacks during the day if you eat during the feeding hours. **Yes, you are going to be hungry.**

It is impossible to say precisely how your body feels during the early stages of intermittent fasting. However, certain things commonly happen to most people when they start intermittent fasting. If you are used to eating 5 to 6 times a day, these effects may be more significant than if you were already eating three meals a day with minimal snacking.

As your body adjusts to intermittent fasting, you will usually feel hungry and hungry.

It is often mental or emotional hunger rather than physical hunger. You may also experience headaches, low energy, and irritability. You may feel a little dizzy, weak, or dizzy while standing.

The severity of these symptoms can change depending on several factors, including your previous diet, but it shouldn't be too dull and should decrease in about a week. **Your body will stabilize.**

After the initial adjustment period, your blood sugar and insulin levels begin to stabilize, and you will start to enjoy the benefits of intermittent fasting. One of the first things you will likely notice is the increase in energy.

You can feel sustained energy throughout the day; instead of feeling awake and productive in the morning, but after being struck by this dreaded afternoon collapse around 2 or 3 p.m., you will feel constant energy. Your blood sugar does not increase or decrease as you do when you eat several meals during the day.

CHAPTER 8:

FAST DAY COOKING TIPS

TIPS FOR A FAST DAY COOKING

1. Increase the amount of low-calorie, low-GI leafy vegetables listed here. Green vegetables are difficult to eat and should be purchased a bit earlier if large quantities are needed. Stir-fried vegetables are delicious. It is best to steam lightly. Invest in a tiered bamboo steamer to promote health and cook protein and vegetables at various stages that are environmentally friendly.

2. Some vegetables will benefit from cooking, but other vegetables should be eaten raw. Cooking certain vegetables, such as carrots, spinach, mushrooms, asparagus, cabbage, and peppers, destroys cell structure without destroying vitamins, allowing them to absorb more food. Mandolin makes the preparation of raw vegetables quick and easy.

3. Fasting days should be low in fat and not fat-free. A teaspoon of olive oil can be used for cooking or sprinkled on vegetables to add flavor. Or use an edible oil spray to get a thin film. The plan includes fatty meats like nuts and pork. Add a light oil dressing to the salad. This means that you are more likely to ingest fat-soluble vitamins.

4. Lemon or orange dressing acids are said to absorb more iron from lush greens such as spinach and kale. Watercress and orange are a great combination with a small number of sesame seeds and sunflower seeds or blanching almonds interspersed with a small amount of protein and crunch.

5. Cook in a pan to reduce high-calorie fats. If the food sticks, splash the water.

6. Weigh the food after cooking for an accurate calorie count.

7. Dairy products are also included. Choose low-fat cheese and skim milk, avoid high-fat yogurt, and choose a low-fat alternative. Drop the latte and throw the butter on a simple day. These are calorie traps.

8. Similarly, avoid starchy white carbohydrates (bread, potatoes, pasta) and instead choose low GI carbohydrates such as vegetables, legumes, and slow-burning cereals. Choose brown rice and quinoa. Use oatmeal for breakfast longer than regular grains.

9. Make sure your fast contains fiber. Eat apples and pears, eat oats for breakfast, and add leafy vegetables.

10. Similarly, avoid starchy white carbohydrates (bread, potatoes, pasta) and instead choose low GI carbohydrates like vegetables, legumes, and slow-burning cereals. Choose brown rice and quinoa. Breakfast porridge stays full longer than standard grain.

11. Be sure to include fiber in your fasting. Eat apples and pears, prepare oats for breakfast, and add leafy

greens.

12. If possible, add flavors. Chili flakes kick a delicious dish. Balsamic vinegar gave acidity. We also add fresh herbs - they are practically calorie-free but give the plate its personality.

13. If you eat protein, you stay longer. Stick to low-fat proteins, including some nuts and legumes. Remove meat skins and fats before cooking.

14. Soup on a hungry day can be a savior, especially if you choose a light soup with leafy greens (Vietnamese Pho is ideal, but keep the noodles low). Soup is a great way to consume the ingredients that you are fed up with and that you struggle within the fridge.

15. If desired, use agave as a sweetener. Lower GI.

IMPROVED APPETITE

When you were pregnant, you probably were suddenly hungry for some of the weirdest things you could think of. These cravings are a mix of psychology and physiology.

When you become pregnant, your body connects you to a new life. This new life requires all original parts and gets building blocks from my host mother. Sometimes the host does not have what it needs and sends the brain a sense of interpretation. The brain interprets this demand as a desire, and the body begins to look for a source of this nutrient.

However, that is just one step. The second step is for the brain to interpret what the body needs. To do this, look at the memory of past foods and search for foods that contain what you need. Knowing where its ingredients are can make your brain feel like eating this food.

This process of identifying the body's needs on different days is confusing, especially when processed foods are added to the mix or a lot of waste is added to the body. The best place for good nutrition is when your child is in the womb and when it is born. What the mother eats goes straight to the child, and this is a great way to get the child on the best possible diet.

If we eat for pleasure and if we eat processed foods, we cannot find a type of food that contains a healthy amount of the nutrients that we need. Therefore, you need to recognize your body with the right diet, without the massive amounts of sugar that are common in modern processed foods. When the body is reintroduced to a better source of dense nutrients, it builds a new library of nutrient information and a library that is available to the body when certain nutrients are needed.

TASTE AND INTERMITTENT FASTING

This is a delicate issue for most people, but a week's preparation should solve it. That's how we are affected by taste and need to protect our taste buds.

Initially, the taste is not just fun. Preference can choose the food you need, which is said to provide nutrition with your body needs.

Taste means appetite, and appetite determines what you eat. When your body needs a particular nutrient, it gives you a desire to look for and consume foods that contain that nutrient. It does not matter if you are a vegan of a lifetime, but if you are new to veganism, you have an appetite for something that's not on the menu. The mechanism is as follows.

When you are a child, your parents will introduce you to foods that are part of your culture and upbringing. If you are in English, you get Bangers and Mash for breakfast. Mexicans get tortillas and quesadillas, and Americans call muesli and toast. It is what you grew up on (I know it is much more than that - it is just an example).

When you consume a particular set of foods, your body records and links different foods with different experiences, for example, if you had sunflower seeds with cereals in the morning, your body will record all of the nutrition you got from sunflower seeds by taking this vitamin E recipe.

From then on, when your body lacks vitamin E, your body unwittingly has an appetite for sunflower seeds. It gives you a desire for the taste of sunflower seeds and the relationship it has in your brain between the need for vitamin E and the preference of sunflower seeds.

Taste is essential to our ability to keep ourselves healthy and replenish what we need when we need it. It is necessary to protect the foods we eat and not be satisfied with aromatic foods. Starting an intermittent fasting lifestyle increases your sense of taste and your desire for what you need, not what you are addicted to. It enables you to let them know that the food they usually crave is no longer available. In this way, we prepared the mind and body of the first week to rely on taste as a guide for choosing the foods as needed.

What does that mean for you? Well, it saves you from

eating unnecessary calories and gaining excessive weight. It works this way. When you want vitamin E from sunflower seeds, instead of picking natural sunflower seeds, you'll want to choose processed and salted ones. Salt appeals to my taste, and it creates habits, but the processed grains are low in vitamin E, and to get the vitamin E, I take more seeds to make up for the deficiency. This leads to higher calorie intake and gives me unnecessary extra weight.

So, apart from seasoning and taste, if you can choose the exact food source of the nutrients you need is the taste. You can find the most natural one you can see in this week of preparation and until the week of the Housewarming. Choosing foods will be clean, and your appetite will accurately reflect what your body needs to replenish.

Remember that intermittent fasting is a lifestyle change that we have to be used to. So, do not consider this a diet, and a week cannot bring you back to your old lifestyle. This is a change in the primary way of looking at you and understanding the senses. It is the direct way to use your natural fat-burning cycle. It is the natural way in which the human body grows.

FOOD TO RETHINK

There are no food groups that needed to be thought over, but the ones that catch the eyes out are the tasty side dishes. Stay away from them at all costs. Taste affects the taste, and its effects affect your food choice and frequency of consumption.

Eating a healthy diet will not only make you hungry in a few hours but will also allow you to work for 1-2 days without refueling. If you find that you cannot get away from the taste, you need to do more.

Therefore, the foods that will be reconsidered are foods that offer flavors such as packaged potato chips and dips, spices, and flavorful side dishes and snacks. An easy way to classify them is to find all pre-packaged and processed foods. After caring for and cleaning your palate, enjoy all the fruits, nuts, vegetables, and seeds available. I do not consume fake meat or fake milk-I know what's made from soy and other non-animal ingredients, but I'm trying to mimic the taste of dairy and meat. That's what you do.

The key to a successful intermittent fasting lifestyle is to change two things in your food efforts. The first is to remove the familiar elements from the food. In this case, we are talking about foods we eat for taste, not nutrition. The second is to change the way with which the taste buds are used to. Using taste buds to select the foods your body needs will increase your health and vitality.

In a week of preparation, there are some things you need to accomplish. First of all, you need to think about the food you eat and why you eat it. There is nothing wrong with eating food for pleasure, as long as you can prevent it enough to distract you from choosing the right food based on taste. As a vegan, we have minimized most of the problems, but by adopting this new lifestyle, we can get rid of the confusion that the taste has to face. There is something like a healthy snack. If not, it is a matter of mindset. Junk food is not nutritious. That's not real Fruit and vegetables with the right mix of herbs and spices in the right amount are pleasant and healthy. Eating what your body needs is happier than eating junk food. This is one of the advantages of intermittent fasting. You can start to hear your body's needs more clearly, and if you give what you need, you will enjoy eating more than chemically flavored junk food.

This is a thing most epicureans do not recognize. Eating can be a fun experience if you eat temporarily and give the body what it is looking for. Eating only out of habit lacks the essential element of nutrition: the need for it.

After all additional flavors and addictive substances have been avoided and the preparation week is over, the palate is cleaned, and you are almost ready to start the start week from day zero (do not worry. Will be explained later). Ideally, it would be great to be able to leave for that. If you can spend a weekend, go to the mountains, go to the beach, work with someone who supports you, or go alone, your Zero Day will be more effective.

HOW TO CHOOSE ZERO-DAY?

There are three things to consider when choosing Zero Day. Remember that Zero Day is the day that begins the first full period of fasting. So, I want to pick it on days when you do not work or when you go to the snack bar or for lunch. You want to get away from this routine, so find a day when you can get away from work and everyday life.

If you can turn off the weekend, you can usually start on a Friday night and spend a Saturday in the wild or in a new place you've never visited before. Some students go to ranches in western California and to mountain monasteries in northern California to escape everyday life and experience not only a zero-day but also a fast. It will give you a whole new meaning. The second thing you have to consider is whether you want to try and do the challenge of dealing with your current routine, or do you want all the help you can get. If you are going to challenge, stay exactly where you are and head for the cold turkey. But if you need all the help you can get, go on a trip somewhere.

Finally, the third thing to consider (which depends on gender) is whether you are at a particular time in your menstrual cycle. If you are ovulating or menstruating, this is not the best time to start a zero-day.

Intermittent fasting lifestyle that you have seen so far is a week of periodic fasting induction designed to transform your body and act as a buffer between your old and your new lifestyle. You cannot help but do what you do every day for the past ten years, 20 years, 30 years or more. Also, expect your body to do well. This is the goal of the introductory week. It introduces your body to intermittent fasting.

But that concludes our introductory week - what's the next step? Well, now, you start your typical day. On regular days, you have two options to choose from. One does intense training, and the others do light exercise. Which one you choose depends on your goals. It depends on whether you plan to sculpt your body or whether you are concentrating heavily on a lot of energy. Overview after induction

The best way to fast intermittently is to go through fast cycles of celebration and fasting. While the Induction Week has allowed you to explore and use your resting metabolic pathway, this section will increase the switching speed between your regular metabolism and your fat-burning metabolism.

If you are a marathon runner, you know what it is like to move from normal metabolism (where you burn calories from foods you eat) to lean metabolism (where you burn stored fat for energy). This is what marathon runners call hitting the wall. When you have calories in your stomach and start the marathon, you come to a point where you exhaust them, and you come to the end of exhaustion. It takes a while for the body to rock and burn fat, and you know the body is rocking because, at that point, you feel like you cannot go on and want to stop. Then you see the athletes slow down, and you can see the immense pain on their faces. Then they get their second wind, and the energy comes back, and they pick up speed again. Why the second wind?

Because his body just changed fuel. Most athletes train long hours not only to increase their speed and efficiency but also to deduce the time they spend when they are off when the body goes on to burn fat. What we did during the initial week was the opportunity to go online. With the 36-hour initial week and the 12-hour preceding week, you have trained your body to move faster. As you enter the real week and increase the pace and frequency to eighteen on and six off, you will find that your body will reach the increased rate, and your switching rate will improve soon. When this happens, you will find that once you eat, the body obediently gets its energy from the food you have just eaten and quickly goes on to burn fat during the 18 hours of fasting. It is an effective system that allows you to shed weight, keep it off, and have an abundance of energy - and what's best is that you will develop a habit for it very soon. This allows you to more easily switch to a lifestyle instead of an unmotivated forced train.

DAILY SWITCHING

During the day-to-day transition, we change our entire routine, so we spend a little of our time focusing on food and the rest of our time on other productive activities.

This is a daily breakdown of 16-8, which means fasting 16 hours a day, then 8 hours. You can reduce your dietary balance and reflect your lifestyle during these 8 hours. This will increase the return on your lifestyle change investment.

When you get into the habit of doing that, your body will spend 12 hours a day on the fat you eat, even 12 hours a day. It is as ideal as possible. The only difference between the different diets is whether you want intensive training or light training. It depends on the degree of your diet.

DAILY STRATEGY

Your daily strategy begins shortly after the admission week. The starting week ended after 3 hours, so there are 8-hour windows instead of 12-hour windows. It is not that bad a difference. In this window, you have to consider how many meals you need. You can adjust this over time. I know that many people have different metabolic profiles, so I do not want to force this onto a preferred number of meals. Some optimize for only three large meals. Whatever you choose, you have to follow it.

1. The intensity of the meals should be a descending profile - that is, the second meal in the window should be the largest, then the slightly lower, then the lower and finally the last meal in the window the smallest from all.

    2.   Fast after a light workout with an appetizer, protein shake, or BCAA.

3. Do heavy exercises before eating heavily.

4. Eat your most massive meal after your workout.

   5.   Eat a light meal before closing the meal window. If you do this:

    1.   You convert fat to muscle, and I'm not talking about fleas and cuts. I speak of slim tones.

    2.   When you have more muscle, it takes more energy to support you - it allows you to eat more and burn fatter.

    3.   The more overweight you burn, the more fuel you can let through, and the leaner energy you send to your brain. Remember that energy from fats helps your mind work better. It is sharper and more agile with faster response times and more acute observations.

    4.   When I start the day with a boost in metabolism, I burn energy all day. That's why I put myself in an automatic path to consistent fuel conversion in 3 weeks.

WHAT TO EAT?

1. DO NOT BE AFRAID TO THINK ABOUT YOUR FAVORITE FOOD.

The psychological mechanism called "getting used" - the more people have something, the less it is tied to it - doing the opposite and trying to suppress food thinking is a faulty strategy. Does that mean? Treat food as friends, not as enemies. Eating is not magical, supernatural, or dangerous. Do not make it the hell Normalize it. Just eat.

2. ADD WATER

Find a non-calorie drink that you like, and then swallow it in bulk. Some people swear by herbal tea. Others prefer foamy mineral water to dance on their tongues, but also tap water. Much of our hydration comes from the foods we eat. Therefore, we may need to add additional drinks beyond our usual intake (check your urine; your urine is pale enough). Should be). There is no scientific basis for drinking the recommended eight glasses of water a day, but there are good reasons to continue drinking. A dry mouth is the last, but not the first sign of dehydration. So, act and recognition before your body are dissatisfied. A glass of water is a quick way to stop hunger, at least temporarily. Also, you will no longer confuse your thirst with hunger.

3. DO NOT EXPECT WEIGHT LOSS ON ANY PARTICULAR DAY

If you have a week where your scale does not seem to shift, even if you do not see the numbers falling, consider the health benefits you will get instead. Remember why you are doing this: not only smaller jeans but also the long-term benefits, the generally accepted advantage of intermittent fasting, destroy disease and strengthen the brain. Extend life. Think of it as your body's pension fund.

4. BE WISE, BE CAREFUL, AND STOP IF YOU FEEL WRONG

This strategy must be implemented flexibly and tolerantly.

You can break the rules if you need to. It is not a race to the finish. So be kind to you and be entertaining. Who wants to live longer when life is miserable? You do not want to growl or sweat in a tired life. You want to go dancing, Right?

5. CONGRATULATIONS

A complete fasting day implies potential weight loss and quantifiable health gains. You have already won. Is breakfast important?

The diet tradition has long indicated that breakfast is the most important meal of the day. Missing it in the morning is like leaving your house without a coat. But not always. According to a recent survey, the more breakfast you have, the bigger your lunch (and dinner). This is not surprising, but it does increase the total number of calories for the day. Wait for a quick later. It is up to you, and the pattern you choose may change over time. What can I drink?

Plenty-unless it has actual calorie content. In fact, as with most decisions on a fast diet, the choice is entirely up to you. Drink plenty of water-it calorie-free, actually free, fuller than you think, and avoids upset your thirst because of hunger. In summer, add a round of cucumber or a pinch of lime. Freeze it and smoke the cube. If you want warmth, miso soup is protein-rich, feels like food, and consumes only 84 calories per cup. Vegetable soup does the same trick. If you are having trouble sleeping, one low-calorie hot chocolate can contain less than 40 calories and can calm you down. Calorie-free drinks are best during the day. It is recommended to pour hot water with lemon to get faster. However, it is recommended to add a pinch of mint leaves or cloves, ginger root slices, or lemongrass. If you like herbal teas, try the unusual flavors (licorice and cinnamon, lemongrass and ginger, lavender, rose, and chamomile). Green tea can have good antioxidant properties. Yes, there is no jury. Please drink if you like it.

Black sugar-free tea and coffee on fasting days can be taken. It is okay if you like milk and artificial sweeteners. But remember that milk calories are added. You are trying to extend the time when you are not burning calories.

Fruit juices look healthy, but are generally surprisingly sugary, contain less fiber than whole fruits, and can increase stealth calories without leaving leaves. Commercial smoothies can have a sugar content similar to that of cola, and because they are acidic, they erode the teeth. They are also loaded with calories. If you want a taste, replace the juice and smoothie with very lean liquor. Probably a dash of elderflower with gushing water and lots of ice.

HOW ABOUT ALCOHOL?

Alcoholic drinks are comfortable, but they only offer "empty" calories. A glass of white wine contains about 120, while a can of 550 ml of beer contains 250. If you cannot say no, skip these on fasting days. This is a unique opportunity to reduce your weekly consumption without continuously feeling disadvantaged. Think of it as an alcoholic two days a week.

AND CAFFEINE?

There is growing evidence that drinking coffee far away from guilty pleasure is useful for preventing mental decline, improving heart health, and reducing the risk of liver cancer and stroke. So, if it moves you and keeps you moving every day, keep drinking coffee. It is a useful weapon against boredom in your arsenal, and coffee breaks can comfortably interrupt your day. There is no metabolic reason to avoid caffeine during the fast. However, if you have problems sleeping, limit your intake later in the day. Of course, please drink black. Chocolates not allowed.

Did you know that chocolate bars are hardly organic food, but did you know what a sweet mocha or apple bar can be? Although processed foods tend to have hidden sugars, which are practical, they do not have the nutritional benefits of useful old plants and proteins. Try carrots, celery sticks, hummus, or a few nuts. Always count them in your daily calories (do not cheat).

Even low-calorie, nutritious foods, and habitual snacks are not recommended. Do not overstimulate as this is part of the motivation to exercise your appetite. If your mouth desperately needs attention, give it a drink. Is it possible to get past the early days using a meal exchange?

SHAKE/JUICE?

Many people say that over-the-counter dietary supplement shakes helped them through the first, usually the hardest, week of intermittent fasting. Shaking is probably easier than counting calories, and on a hungry day, you can take a sip when the hungry waves hit. We aren't big fans because we think real food is better. But if you find it useful, definitely try it. It is best to choose a brand with low sugar content. What are the consequences of fraud and some chips or cookies?

For clarity, this is a book about fasting and voluntary

abstention from eating. The reason why this is good for you goes far beyond the fact that you simply eat fewer calories. It occurs because our body is designed for intermittent fasting. Adversity only makes you stronger. While hunger is terrible, a little short, sharp, shocking food restrictions are reasonable.

Your goal is, therefore, to open a food-free breathing space for your body. It does not hurt to reach 510 calories (615 calories for men). Fasting never goes away. The idea of reducing calories by a quarter of your daily intake on a day of fasting has only been clinically proven to have a systemic effect on metabolism. There is no particular "magic" at 500 or 600 calories, but you should stick to these numbers. Specific parameters are required to make a strategy effective in the medium term.

An "extra cookie" on a fasting day is precisely the opposite of your goal (which will likely increase your blood sugar and consume most of your tolerated amount in a butter byte). Needless to say, if you are fasting, you need to think wisely and consistently about your food choices according to the plan outlined here. I will be motivated to exercise, and I will remember that tomorrow is approaching.

WHO ELSE SHOULD NOT FAST?

There are certain groups where fasting is not recommended. People with type 1 diabetes and people with eating disorders are included in this list. If you are already very slim, do not fast. Children should never fast. They are still growing and should not be exposed to any nutritional stress. If you have an underlying disorder, talk to your doctor about how to do it before starting to lose weight.

DO YOU HAVE A HEADACHE?

Doing so may be due to dehydration rather than a lack of calories. A slight withdrawal symptom may appear with sugar (or caffeine if you drop it), but the short fasting is not a particular concern. Continue drinking water. Treat the headache as usual. If you feel a particularly unpleasant fast today, stop it. You are responsible.

DO YOU HAVE TO WORRY ABOUT HYPOGLYCEMIA?

When you are in good health, your body is a very efficient and functioning machine that is used to regulate your blood sugar level effectively. A quick fast is unlikely to cause a hypoglycemic reaction. The recent widespread idea that pasture is necessary to prevent "blood sugar crashes" is a myth. If you eat low GI foods on a fasting day according to the guidelines here, your blood sugar will remain stable. But do not overdo it.

Fasting longer than the recommended biweekly, 24-hour nutritional program here may result in a drop in blood pressure, glucose levels, and dizziness. So be quick and smart. If you have diabetes, consult your doctor before you start changing your diet.

I'M TIRED !!!

Researchers in Illinois hypothesized that on a hungry day, subjects would feel "less and less physically active." Like everyday life, you have a few days up and down, good days and bad days. As an example, many of the intermittent fasting we encountered reports a surge in energy rather than exhaustion. How's it going? Early days may end earlier than usual-not drinking alcohol, and getting enough sleep is an excellent way to have breakfast first.

HOWEVER, DO I SLEEP HUNGRY?

Probably not, but it depends on your particular metabolism and how you measure your calorie consumption in the early morning. If you are hungry, please be careful. Bubble bath, a good book, stretching, and herbal tea adds psychology. Congratulations on the end of the next day of fasting. Surprisingly, the fasting people may report that even if the alarm sounds, they won't run into the fridge without waking up violently. Hunger is a subtle animal, and your appetite will soon find its rhythm.

WILL, MY BODY GO INTO HUNGER MODE AND CONTINUES TO GET FAT?

You do not limit your calories every day, so your body never goes into the legendary hunger mode. Your fasting is never intense. Your body burns energy from fat stores but does not consume muscle tissue because it is always conservative and short-lived. Studies have shown that occasional fasting does not suppress metabolism.

Intermittent fasting also does not increase the level of the hunger-stimulating hormone ghrelin. Researchers at the Pennington Centre for Biomedical Research in Louisiana found that "ghrelin remained unchanged after 36 hours of fasting in both men and women". A licensed path to health and well-being.

WHAT IF EVERYONE AROUND ME EATS ONE OF MY FASTING DAYS?

Get involved, but with a calm conscience. While support from family and friends is beneficial, you will only feel confident when you compose a song and dance on your fast. Diet becomes an obstacle that should integrate happily and calmly into your life. Think of your asset: you will generally eat again tomorrow. Of course, some days are more difficult than others. According to Varady among his subjects, hunger increased by the eighth week: "We think it may have happened because this week of study corresponded to Memorial Day weekend and the issues may have had hungry when they participated in culinary festivities."

If you know you have a social event - or food celebration - in the newspaper, fast the night before or the next day. The flexibility of the plan explicitly means - in fact, it requires - that you always go to this wedding, anniversary, birthday dinner, baptism, bar mitzvah, dinner, chic restaurant. Take a break for Christmas, Easter, Thanksgiving, and Diwali. Yes, you could gain some weight, but it is a life, not a life sentence. You can get around at any time, eat fries and dips and stuff on sticks, and then return to a more difficult fast after the party ends.

WHAT IF I AM CURRENTLY OBESE?

Clinical studies have shown that intermittent fasting is a lasting - if not one of the most effective - way for overweight people to lose weight and keep it off. The bigger you are, the more critical your initial weight loss will be. If you are overweight, traditional restrictive diets have likely failed for some reason. The fast diet is distinguished from the "stimulants" on non-fast days by its flexibility, guilt war, and expresses approval.

Illinois studies have shown that overweight people can

adapt quickly to ADF. They were able to remain physically active despite the fast. In summary, "overweight and obese patients experience significant improvements in regimens." As with any underlying disease, we recommend that you fast under supervision. Should I add a third day if I want to see accelerated results? There is no reason not to do it; after all, this is what Dr. Krista Varady's Alternate Day Fasters (ADF) do. However, pay attention to rapid fatigue.

One of the keys to success is that fast nutrition only requires short-term engagement. Ask your body to do more than that, and it can sit up and refuse to behave, making the recommended fasting program more difficult. Experience has shown us that two days are enough. But if you have a date and little party pants on standby, one occasional sneaky day shouldn't hurt. However, do not try an intensive long-term diet. It is not worth it unless you are obese and under medical supervision.

CONCLUSION

How we do what our mind, body, and spirit are and howfood is consumed by our watches, not when it is currently needed or when our body needs it. I saw how it evolved. Strangely, the ancestors of the cave decided to go out and look for lunch when they saw the sun hanging over the zenith. It didn't work that way.

Our body has grown accustomed to the planned meal. As food became part of our itinerary, so did our habits. Their eating habits were particularly useful in making room for organized work schedules. But they made no sense for our health or our lives.

The evidence-based diet review shows that the bottom line is trying to adjust intake but still keeps the frame in the context of a three-meal day. We are looking at the opportunity to cut fat, the chance to cut carbohydrates, and even talk about cutting the candy. But the problem is that it is all based on the dietary conditions that we know.

Food is no longer the natural source of energy that we have developed. Food has been processed for taste and convenience, stored for packaging, and colored for appeal. Food is no longer food. It is a set of marketing principles. Therefore, we know that our bodies adapt and that the long-term effects include illness and a regular diet. We are entering this cycle of unhealthy outcomes.

Doing these two things can increase the power of intermittent fasting.

1. Remove all highly processed foods from your diet and replace them with organic and natural foods.

2. Turn most of your diet into nutritious and should be part of your weekly diet. In the lights of food items like kale, garlic, ginger, Nora + fermented product, all types of berries and leafy vegetables can turn the course of effects in the diet.

Intermittent fasting is a powerful tool. Changing biology and psychology. For most people, the fasting process is mentally more challenging than physically limiting. By accepting intermittent fasting, they suddenly remove the restraint of their indoctrination and see the value of life in its original sense.

Welcome to a happy fast and a new you.

DELICIOUS RECIPES

SPICY CHOCOLATE FAT BOMBS

READY IN: 8mins
SERVES: 24
INGREDIENTS

2/3 cup coconut oil
2/3 cup smooth peanut butter
1/2 cup dark cocoa
4 (6 g) packets stevia (or to taste)
1 tablespoon ground cinnamon
1/4 teaspoon kosher salt
1/2 cup toasted coconut flakes
1/4 teaspoon cayenne (to taste)

DIRECTIONS

Combine coconut oil, peanut butter, and cocoa powder in a double boiler set over a pot of simmering water. Heat, whisking, until melted and smooth.
Add stevia, cinnamon, and salt and stir to combine.
Divide mixture among a silicone mini muffin tray. (Alternatively, line a mini muffin tin with liners and divide mixture among liners.).
Top with coconut and cayenne and transfer to freezer until firm, about 30 minutes.

Nadia Wilmots

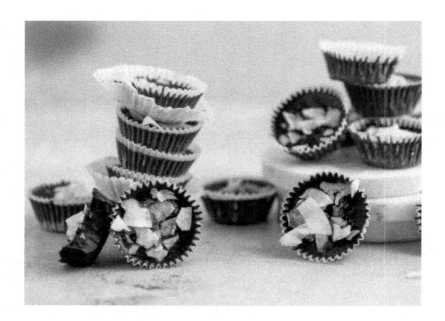

AVOCADO QUESADILLAS

READY IN: 31mins
SERVES: 2
INGREDIENTS

2   vine-ripe tomatoes, seeded and chopped into 1/4 inch pieces
1   ripe avocado, peeled, pitted, and chopped into 1/4 inch pieces
1   tablespoon chopped red onion
2   teaspoons fresh lemon juice
1/4   teaspoon Tabasco sauce
salt and pepper
1/4   cup sour cream
3   tablespoons chopped fresh coriander
24   inches flour tortillas
1/2   teaspoon vegetable oil
1 1/3   cups shredded monterey jack cheese

DIRECTIONS

In a small bowl, mix together the tomatoes, avocado, onion, lemon juice and Tabasco.
Season to taste with salt and pepper.
In another small bowl, mix together sour cream, coriander, salt and pepper to taste.
Put tortillas on a baking sheet and brush tops with oil.
Broil tortillas 2 to 4 inches from heat until pale golden.
Sprinkle tortillas evenly with cheese and broil until cheese is melted.
Spread avocado mixture evenly over 2 tortillas and top each with 1 of remaining tortillas, cheese side down to make 2 quesadillas.
Transfer quesadillas to a cutting board and cut into 4 wedges.
Top each wedge with a dollop of sour cream mixture and serve warm.

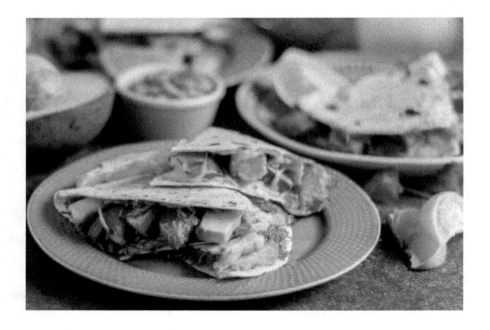

COBB SALAD WITH BROWN DERBY DRESSING

READY IN: 30mins
SERVES: 2
INGREDIENTS

1/2 head iceberg lettuce
1/2 bunch watercress
1 bunch chicory lettuce
1/2 head romaine lettuce
2 medium tomatoes, skinned and seeded
1/2 lb smoked turkey breast
6 slices crisp bacon
1 avocado, sliced in half, seeded and peeled
3 hardboiled egg
2 tablespoons chives, chopped fine
1/2 cup blue cheese, crumbled

DRESSING

2 tablespoons water
1/8 teaspoon sugar
3/4 teaspoon kosher salt
1/2 teaspoon Worcestershire sauce
2 tablespoons balsamic vinegar (or red wine vinegar)
1 tablespoon fresh lemon juice
1/2 teaspoon fresh ground black pepper
1/8 teaspoon Dijon mustard
2 tablespoons olive oil
2 cloves garlic, minced very fine

DIRECTIONS

Chop all the greens very, very fine (almost minced).
Arrange in rows in a chilled salad bowl.
Cut the tomatoes in half, seed, and chop very fine.
Fine dice the turkey, avocado, eggs and bacon.
Arrange all the ingredients, including the blue cheese, in rows across the lettuces.
Sprinkle with the chives.

Present at the table in this fashion, then toss with the dressing at the very last minute and serve in chilled salad bowls.
Serve with fresh french bread.
FOR THE DRESSING: Combine all the ingredients except the olive oil in a blender and blend.
Slowly, with the machine running, add the oil and blend well.
Keep refrigerated.
*NOTE:This dish should be kept chilled, and served as chilled as possible.

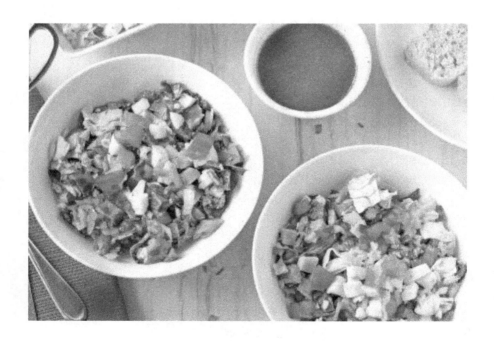

LEMON SALMON

READY IN: 27mins
SERVES: 4
INGREDIENTS

- 2 teaspoons fresh dill
- 1/2 teaspoon pepper
- 1/2 teaspoon salt
- 1/2 teaspoon garlic powder
- 1 1/2 lbs salmon fillets
- 1/4 cup packed brown sugar
- 1 chicken bouillon cube, mixed with
- 3 tablespoons water
- 3 tablespoons oil
- 3 tablespoons soy sauce
- 4 tablespoons finely chopped green onions
- 1 lemon, thinly sliced
- 2 slices onions, seperated into rings

DIRECTIONS

Sprinkle dill, pepper, salt and garlic powder over salmon.
Place in shallow glass pan.
Mix sugar, chicken boullion, oil, soy sauce, and green onions.
Pour over salmon.
Cover and chill for 1 hour, turn once.
Drain and discard marinade.
Put on grill on med heat, place lemon and onion on top.
Cover and cook for 15 minutes, or until fish is done.

Nadia Wilmots

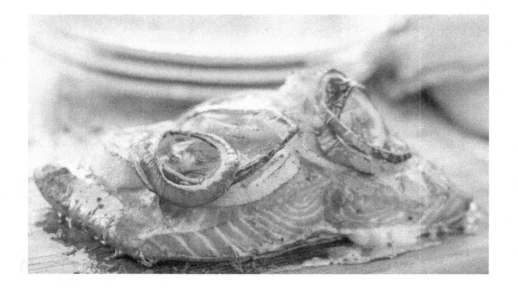

VEGGIE CHEESY CHICKEN SALAD

READY IN: 35mins
SERVES: 1-2
INGREDIENTS

1 cup cooked boneless skinless chicken breast, cubed
1/4 cup celery, finely chopped
1/4 cup carrot, shaved into ribbons
1/2 cup Baby Spinach, roughly chopped
2 1/2 tablespoons fat-free mayonnaise
2 tablespoons nonfat sour cream
1/8 teaspoon dried parsley
2 teaspoons Dijon mustard
1/4 cup reduced-fat sharp cheddar cheese, shredded

DIRECTIONS

Mix all ingredients in a bowl so that everything is coated well with the mayonnaise mixture.
Chill in the fridge for at least 30 minutes but you could do it the night before.
Serve.

Nadia Wilmots

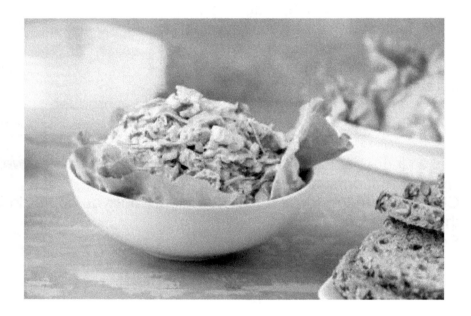

FRIED 'FISH' TACOS

READY IN: 50mins
YIELD: 8 small tacos
INGREDIENTS

14 ounces silken tofu
2 cups panko breadcrumbs
1/2 cup plain flour
1/2 teaspoon salt
1 teaspoon smoked paprika
1/2 teaspoon cayenne pepper
1 teaspoon ground cumin
1/2 cup non-dairy milk
vegetable oil, for frying
1/4 head cabbage, finely shredded
1 ripe avocado
8 small tortillas
vegan mayonnaise, to serve

PICKLED ONION
1 red onion, peeled, finely sliced
1/4 cup apple cider vinegar
1 tablespoon sugar
1 teaspoon salt

DIRECTIONS

Pat the tofu with a fiew pieces of kitchen roll to remove excess moisture. Use a knife to break the tofu into rough 1-inch chunks – I like them to be imperfect, not cubes, so they look nicer!
Place the breadcrumbs into one wide shallow bowl.
Place the flour, salt, smoked paprika, cayenne and cumin into another wide shallow bowl and stir together.
Place the milk into a third wide shallow bowl.
Take the chunks of tofu and gently coat them in the flour then the milk then the breadcrumbs and onto a baking

sheet.
Fill a deep frying pan with 1/2 -inch depth of vegetable oil.

Place over a medium heat and let the oil get hot – sprinkle a breadcrumb in and if it start to bubble and brown, the oil is hot enough. Add chunks of breaded tofu to the oil and fry until golden underneath then flip and cook so it's golden all over. Remove to a baking sheet lined with kitchen roll to drain. Repeat with the remaining tofu.
For the pickled onion:
Heat the apple cide vinegar, salt and sugar in a small pot until steaming. Place the finely sliced red onion in a bowl or jar and pour the hot vinegar over. Let it sit for at least 30 minutes to soften and turn pink.
Serve the hot fried tofu in warmed tortillas (I warm them over the lit gas ring of my stove), pickled onion, a smear of vegan mayo, some avocado and shredded cabbage.

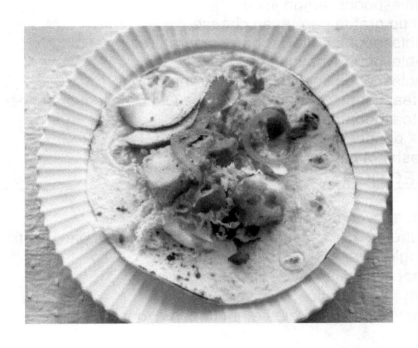

TILAPIA PARMESAN

READY IN: 35mins
SERVES: 4
INGREDIENTS

2 lbs tilapia fillets (orange roughy, cod or red snapper can be substituted)
2 tablespoons lemon juice
1/2 cup grated parmesan cheese
4 tablespoons butter, room temperature
3 tablespoons mayonnaise
3 tablespoons finely chopped green onions
1/4 teaspoon seasoning salt (I like Old Bay seasoning here)
1/4 teaspoon dried basil
black pepper
1 dash hot pepper sauce

DIRECTIONS

Preheat oven to 350 degrees.
In buttered 13-by-9-inch baking dish or jellyroll pan, lay fillets in single layer.
Do not stack fillets.
Brush top with juice.
In bowl combine cheese, butter, mayonnaise, onions and seasonings.
Mix well with fork.
Bake fish in preheated oven 10 to 20 minutes or until fish just starts to flake.
Spread with cheese mixture and bake until golden brown, about 5 minutes.
Baking time will depend on the thickness of the fish you use.
Watch fish closely so that it does not overcook.
Makes 4 servings.
Note: This fish can also be made in a broiler.
Broil 3 to 4 minutes or until almost done.

Add cheese and broil another 2 to 3 minutes or until browned.
Thank you Mama's Supper Club in Wisconsin.

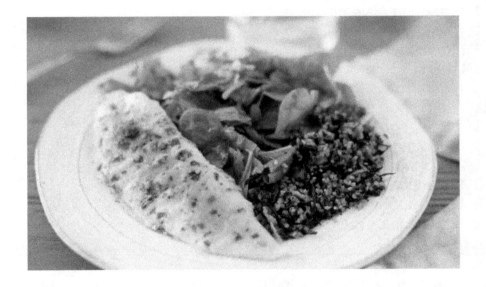

CHICKEN BREASTS WITH AVOCADO TAPENADE

READY IN: 15mins
SERVES: 4
INGREDIENTS

- 4 boneless skinless chicken breast halves
- 1 tablespoon grated lemon peel
- 5 tablespoons fresh lemon juice, divided
- 2 tablespoons olive oil, divided
- 1 teaspoon olive oil, divided
- 1 garlic clove, finely chopped
- 1/2 teaspoon salt
- 1/4 teaspoon ground black pepper
- 2 garlic cloves, roasted and mashed
- 1/2 teaspoon sea salt
- 1/4 teaspoon fresh ground pepper
- 1 medium tomatoes, seeded and finely chopped
- 1/4 cup small green pimento stuffed olive, thinly sliced
- 3 tablespoons capers, rinsed
- 2 tablespoons fresh basil leaves, finely sliced
- 1 large Hass avocado, ripe, finely chopped

DIRECTIONS

In sealable plastic bag, combine chicken and marinade of lemon peel, 2 tablespoons lemon juice, 2 tablespoons olive oil, garlic, salt and pepper. Seal bag and refrigerate for 30 minutes.

In bowl, whisk together remaining 3 tablespoons lemon juice, roasted garlic, remaining 1/2 teaspoons olive oil, sea salt and fresh ground pepper. Mix in tomato, green olives, capers, basil and avocado; set aside.

Remove chicken from bag and discard marinade. Grill over medium-hot coals for 4 to 5 minutes per side or to desired degree of doneness.

Serve with Avocado Tapenade.

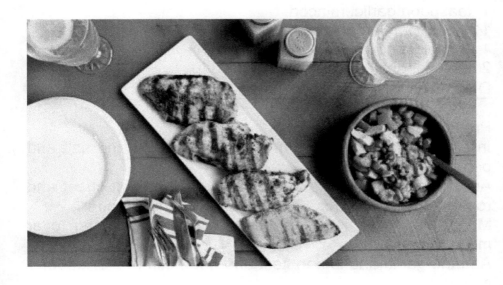

ROASTED BROCCOLI W LEMON GARLIC & PINE NUTS

READY IN: 22mins
SERVES: 4
INGREDIENTS

1 lb broccoli floret
2 tablespoons olive oil
salt & freshly ground black pepper
2 tablespoons unsalted butter
1 teaspoon garlic, minced
1/2 teaspoon lemon zest, grated
1 -2 tablespoon fresh lemon juice
2 tablespoons pine nuts, toasted

DIRECTIONS

Preheat oven to 500 degrees.
In a large bowl, toss the broccoli with the oil and salt and pepper to taste.
Arrange the florets in a single layer on a baking sheet and roast, turning once, for 12 minutes, or until just tender.
Meanwhile, in a small saucepan, melt the butter over medium heat.
Add the garlic and lemon zest and heat, stirring, for about 1 minute.
Let cool slightly and stir in the lemon juice.
Place the broccoli in a serving bowl, pour the lemon butter over it and toss to coat.
Scatter the toasted pine nuts over the top.

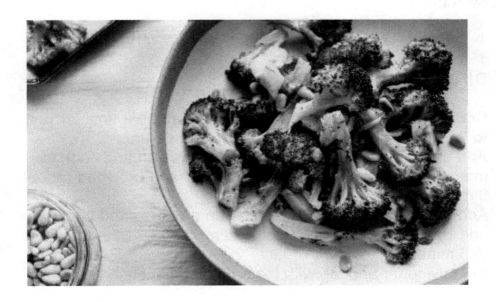

BRUSSELS SPROUTS WITH BACON AND ONIONS

READY IN: 30mins
SERVES: 6
INGREDIENTS

2 slices bacon
1 small yellow onion, thinly sliced
1/4 teaspoon salt (or to taste)
3/4 cup water
1 teaspoon Dijon mustard
1 lb Brussels sprout, trimmed, halved and very thinly sliced
1 tablespoon cider vinegar

DIRECTIONS

Cook bacon in a large skillet over medium heat until crisp (5 to 7 minutes); drain on paper towels, then crumble.
Add onion and salt to the drippings in the pan and cook over medium heat, stirring often, until tender and browned (about 3 minutes).
Add water and mustard, scraping up any browned bits, then add Brussels sprouts and cook, stirring often, until tender (4 to 6 minutes).
Stir in vinegar and top with the crumbled bacon.

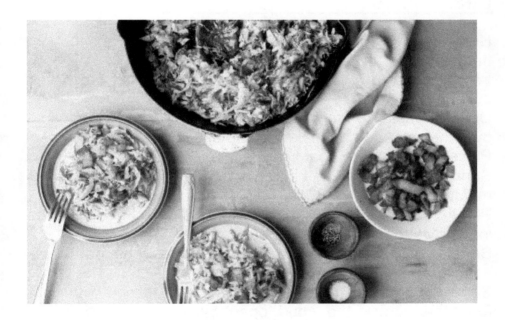

BAKED POTATO

READY IN: 1hr 10mins
SERVES: 1
INGREDIENTS

1 large russet potato
canola oil
kosher salt

DIRECTIONS

Heat oven to 350°F and position racks in top and bottom thirds.
Wash potato (or potatoes) thoroughly with a stiff brush and cold running water.
Dry, then using a standard fork poke 8 to 12 deep holes all over the spud so that moisture can escape during cooking.
Place in a bowl and coat lightly with oil.
Sprinkle with kosher salt and place potato directly on rack in middle of oven.
Place a baking sheet (I put a piece of aluminum foil) on the lower rack to catch any drippings.
Bake 1 hour or until skin feels crisp but flesh beneath feels soft.
Serve by creating a dotted line from end to end with your fork, then crack the spud open by squeezing the ends towards one another.
It will pop right open.
But watch out, there will be some steam.
NOTE: If you're cooking more than 4 potatoes, you'll need to extend the cooking time by up to 15 minutes.

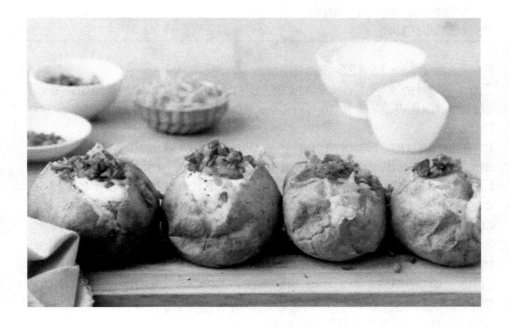

CAULIFLOWER POPCORN

READY IN: 1hr 10mins
SERVES: 4
INGREDIENTS

1 head cauliflower or 1 head equal amount of pre-cut commercially prepped cauliflower
4 tablespoons olive oil
1 teaspoon salt, to taste

DIRECTIONS

Preheat oven to 425 degrees.
Trim the head of cauliflower, discarding the core and thick stems; cut florets into pieces about the size of ping-pong balls.
In a large bowl, combine the olive oil and salt, whisk, then add the cauliflower pieces and toss thoroughly.
Line a baking sheet with parchment for easy cleanup (you can skip that, if you don't have any) then spread the cauliflower pieces on the sheet and roast for 1 hour, turning 3 or 4 times, until most of each piece has turned golden brown.
(The browner the cauliflower pieces turn, the more caramelization occurs and the sweeter they'll taste).
Serve immediately and enjoy!
Where I got it: I originally heard about this recipe at Gail's Recipe Swap, where Josh posted it and many folks tried and loved it.

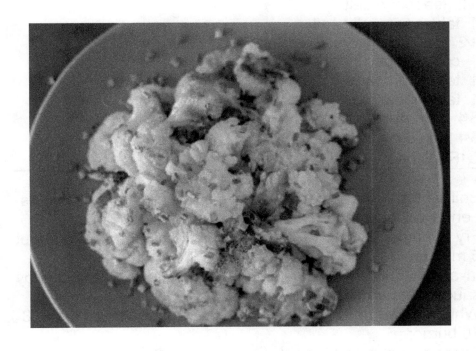

LENTIL BURGERS

READY IN: 1hr 10mins
YIELD: 8-10 burgers
INGREDIENTS

1 cup dry lentils, well rinsed
2 1/2 cups water
1/2 teaspoon salt
1 tablespoon olive oil
1/2 medium onion, diced
1 carrot, diced
1 teaspoon pepper
1 tablespoon soy sauce
3/4 cup rolled oats, finely ground
3/4 cup breadcrumbs

DIRECTIONS

Boil lentils in the water with the salt for around 45 minutes. Lentils will be soft and most of the water will be gone.
Fry the onions and carrot in the oil until soft, it will take about 5 minutes.
In a bowl mix the cooked ingredients with the pepper, soy sauce, oats and bread cumbs.
While still warm form the mixture into patties, it will make 8-10 burgers.
Burgers can then be shallow fried for 1-2 minutes on each side or baked at 200C for 15 minutes.

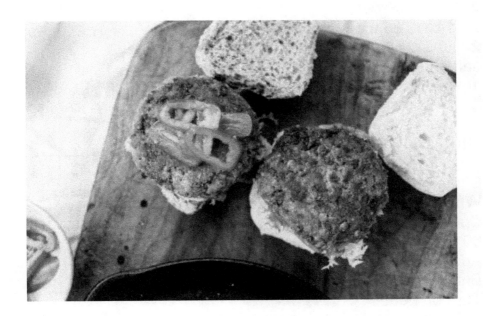

BLACK BEAN SOUP

READY IN: 25mins
SERVES: 4
INGREDIENTS

- 3 tablespoons olive oil
- 1 medium onion, chopped
- 1 tablespoon ground cumin
- 2 -3 cloves garlic
- 2 (14 1/2 ounce) cans black beans
- 2 cups chicken broth or 2 cups vegetable broth
- salt and pepper
- 1 small red onion, chopped fine
- 1/4 cup cilantro, coarsely chopped or finely chopped (whatever you prefer)

DIRECTIONS

Saute onion in olive oil.
When onion becomes translucent, add cumin.
Cook 30 seconds, then add garlic and cook for another 30 to 60 seconds.
Add 1 can black beans and 2 cups vegetable broth.
Bring to a simmer, stirring occasionally.
Turn off heat.
Using a hand blender, blend the ingredients in the pot, or transfer to a blender.
Add the second can of beans to the pot along with blended ingredients and bring to a simmer.
Serve soup with bowls of red onion and cilantro for garnish.
I add a bit of cilantro to the pot, too.
Can be doubled or frozen.

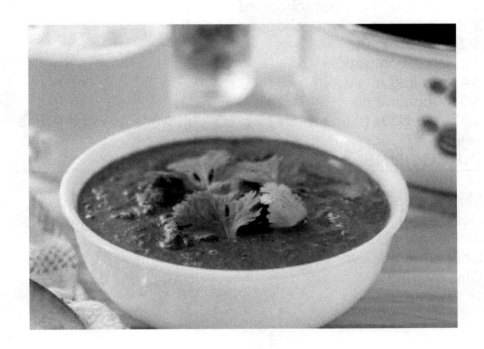

SAUERKRAUT SALAD

READY IN: 15mins
SERVES: 6
INGREDIENTS

1 (1 lb) can sauerkraut, drained but not rinsed
1 cup celery, chopped fine
1/2 cup green pepper, chopped fine
2 tablespoons onions, chopped fine
1/2 teaspoon salt
1/2 teaspoon pepper
3/4 cup sugar
1/3 cup salad oil
1/3 cup cider (I use white) or 1/3 cup white vinegar (I use white)

DIRECTIONS

Mix chopped vegetables with sauerkraut.
Heat sugar, oil, vinegar, salt, and pepper over low heat just until sugar dissolves.
Cool and pour over vegetables.
Chill overnight.

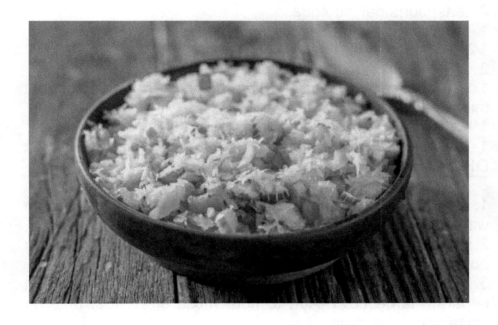

COCONUT KEFIR BANANA MUFFINS

READY IN: 45mins
SERVES: 12
INGREDIENTS

2 cups all-purpose flour
1 cup granulated sugar
1 cup unsweetened dried shredded coconut
2 teaspoons baking soda
1 teaspoon baking powder
1/2 teaspoon salt
2 ripe bananas, mashed
1 1/2 cups pc dairy-free kefir probiotic fermented coconut milk
1/4 cup cold-pressed liquid coconut oil
1 teaspoon vanilla extract

DIRECTIONS

1. Preheat oven to 350°F (180°C). Mist 12-count muffin tin with cooking spray. Set aside.
2. Whisk together flour, sugar, coconut, baking soda, baking powder and salt in large bowl. Set aside.
3. Whisk together bananas, kefir, coconut oil and vanilla in separate large bowl. Add to flour mixture; stir just until no white streaks remain.
4. Divide among the wells of prepared muffin tin. Bake until tops are golden and toothpick inserted in centres comes out clean; about 30 minutes. Let cool in muffin tin for 15 minutes.

Chef's tip: To freeze muffins, let them cool completely on a rack, then transfer to an airtight container or resealable freezer bag and freeze for up to one month. For extra protection against freezer burn, you can wrap the muffins individually in plastic wrap or foil before placing in the container or bag. Thaw muffins in the fridge overnight or microwave straight from frozen until warmed through; about 20 to 30 seconds.

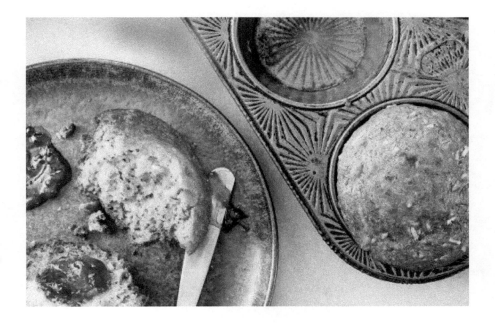

CPSIA information can be obtained
at www.ICGtesting.com
Printed in the USA
LVHW011645130621
690126LV00014B/989